The Rosedale Diet

the Rosedale diet

RON ROSEDALE, M.D.,
and CAROL COLMAN

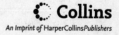

Collins
An Imprint of HarperCollinsPublishers

DISCLAIMER

This book is written as a source of information only. The information
contained in this book should by no means be considered a
substitute for the advice of a qualified medical professional,
who should always be consulted before beginning any
new diet, exercise, or other health program.
All efforts have been made to ensure the accuracy of the information
contained in this book as of the date published. The author and
the publisher expressly disclaim responsibility for any adverse
effects arising from the use or application of the
information contained herein.

PRIVACY DISCLAIMER

The names of the individuals discussed in this book
have been changed to protect their privacy.

THE ROSEDALE DIET. Copyright © 2004 by Ron Rosedale and Carol Colman.
All rights reserved. Printed in the United States of America. No part of this book
may be used or reproduced in any manner whatsoever without written permission
except in the case of brief quotations embodied in critical articles and reviews.
For information address HarperCollins Publishers, 10 East 53rd Street,
New York, NY 10022.

HarperCollins books may be purchased for educational, business, or sales
promotional use. For information please write: Special Markets Department,
HarperCollins Publishers, 10 East 53rd Street, New York, NY 10022.

First Collins paperback edition published 2005.

Designed by Ellen Cipriano

Library of Congress Cataloging-in-Publication Data

Rosedale, Ron.
    The Rosedale diet/Ron Rosedale and Carol Colman.—1st ed.
        p.   cm.
    Includes bibliographical references and index.
    ISBN 0-06-056572-1 (hc)
    1. Reducing diets.   2. Weight loss.   I. Colman, Carol.   II. Title.

    RM222.2.R6473   2004
    613.2'5—dc22   2004045356
ISBN 0-06-056573-X (pbk.)

        05 06 07 08 09 WB/RRD 10 9 8 7 6 5 4 3 2 1

To my parents, my sisters, and my son
for their love and support

RON ROSEDALE

···Contents

⋯ ▪ ▪ ▪ Acknowledgments

First and foremost, we'd like to thank Toni Sciarra for her superb editing of this book, and for stepping in and taking over the project in midstream. We'd also like to thank Nicholas Darrell for all of his help, Megan Newman for her support and vision, and the wonderful production and publicity teams at HarperCollins for their hard work. Without all of them, this book would never have become a reality. Many thanks to Jeremiah Stamler, M.D., professor emeritus, Department of Preventive Medicine at Northwestern University Medical School, who encouraged Ron's interest in the strong relationship between diet and heart disease, and to Gary Spoleta for his unwavering support for this project. We'd also like to extend our gratitude to Jena Latham for her fabulous recipes, and Peggy Dace for all of her help. A special thanks to our agent, Richard Curtis, who has so ably represented Carol for more than two decades, and for launching Ron on his career as an author.

The Rosedale Diet

Everything You Need to Know About the Rosedale Diet

chapter one

Get Slim, Live Longer, Be Healthier

Want a slim, sculpted body and a longer life? There's a tried and true way to achieve both. Eating less . . . a lot less. Decades ago, researchers discovered that if you put laboratory animals on a very low calorie diet—about one-third fewer calories than normal—they can live up to *two times longer* than well-fed animals. Not surprisingly, food-restricted animals retain their sleek, youthful figures. What is truly amazing, however, is that their bodies not only appear younger, but by every objective laboratory measure, *they are younger*. Levels of key hormones that normally fluctuate with age, and other important markers of aging remain remarkably stable. Nor do food-restricted animals suffer as often from the chronic diseases associated with "normal" aging, such as diabetes, heart disease, and cancer.

Slim for life. Healthy for life. A *longer* life in a "younger" body. Despite these wonderful results, no one is seriously suggesting that humans should follow such a punishing diet. Who wants to starve? Who willingly can?

The fact is, you don't have to starve to be in great shape or to enjoy the prospect of a longer, disease-free life. Thanks to the Rosedale Diet, you can have all the benefits of a strict, low calorie diet—a great body, great health, and the promise of longevity—without ever having to feel a hunger pang.

The even better news is that you can lose weight and get healthy while still eating delicious meals and snacks such as chicken tortillas, wraps, guacamole, nuts (even so-called fattening nuts like macadamia nuts), lobster salad, raspberry cheesecake, and eggs Benedict. No starving. No hunger. The best part of all is that you will be back in control of your hunger, your weight, and your life.

My program has worked for thousands of my patients, and it can work for you. By following the Rosedale Diet, my patients have not only successfully lost weight, but have rejuvenated their bodies and reclaimed their health. The once obese are now trim and fit, in an amazingly short period of time. Remarkably, the same biomarkers of longevity seen in calorie-restricted animals are seen in my patients. In fact, by every objective laboratory measure, my patients have "de-aged" their bodies:

- High blood sugar levels, a hallmark of aging, fall to normal, healthy levels.
- Body temperature stays lower in my patients, a sign that their bodies are running more efficiently.
- Key hormones are restored to more youthful levels.
- High blood lipid levels (triglycerides) plummet to a healthy range.

The so-called diseases of aging, such as type 2 diabetes, a veritable epidemic among people over forty, and heart disease, the number one killer of both men and women, are vastly improved. In fact, after following my program for a few weeks, my patients are able to throw out most of their prescription medicines.

My patients not only look great, but they tell me that they feel great too, and have a huge amount of energy. The best news is, unlike calorie-restricted animals who are kept in cages and starved to enjoy these benefits, my patients feel full and satisfied. It's too early to say whether my patients will live longer—we need to wait another thirty or forty years for that data—but all indications are that they will. I can say with certainty that the *quality* of their lives is significantly better. (My patients can speak for themselves, and they do. They tell their own stories in their own words, throughout this book.)

Within this book, you will find the tools that you need to take back control of your weight, and ultimately, your life. You will be empowered with the latest scientific information on how to lose weight safely, quickly, and permanently. Once you start the Rosedale Diet, you, too, can experience the same spectacular success in terms of both weight loss and better health enjoyed by my patients.

■ GETTING TO THE HEART OF OBESITY

The Rosedale Diet works because it corrects the underlying metabolic aberration at the root cause of both obesity and premature aging: hormonal dysfunction. Hormones are chemical messengers that direct all body activities, including how much you eat, and ultimately, whether you are fat or fit. Your hormones can work for you or against you. The wrong diet creates hormonal imbalances that trigger hunger and food cravings, the main problems that prevent people from losing weight and keeping it off. The right diet—the Rosedale Diet—almost magically controls hunger and eliminates food cravings. That is why it works so well.

Hunger is a powerful force. As I tell my patients, following a diet while trying to fight hunger is like trying to hold on to the edge of a cliff and hoping that gravity will go away. Eventually, you're going to let go. If you're hungry, eventually you're going to eat and chances are, you'll overeat to make up for lost time.

How does my diet curb hunger? The Rosedale Diet is specially designed to control the key hormone that regulates both appetite and weight loss. That hormone is *leptin*. Leptin is produced by your fat cells. It tells your brain when to eat, how much to eat and most important, when to *stop* eating. Leptin is also critical for many of the body's most important functions, including the regulation of blood circulation, the prevention of blood clots, making new bone, regulation of body temperature, and reproduction. In fact, if a woman produces too little leptin, she will stop menstruating, and therefore will be unable to conceive. Very recently, leptin amazed the scientific community when it was found to be able to rewire critical and central portions of the brain to better do its bidding. The more scientists research leptin, the more they learn about how vital it is to life.

As hormones go, leptin is the new kid on the block. In fact, it's so new, most of your doctors may not have heard of it, or are unsure what it does. Yet, I consider leptin to be so important for the health and well-being of my patients that I always measure their leptin levels, and if I have any say in the matter, doing so will become standard medical practice within a few years. Measuring leptin is easy—it's a simple blood test—but it tells me volumes about my patients' potential for gaining weight and the ease with which they will be able to shed excess pounds. Blood leptin levels indicate how well leptin is functioning in your body. High fasting levels of leptin (from blood taken after waking and before eating breakfast) mean that leptin is not functioning well, and therefore, unless leptin is brought down to a healthy level, losing weight and keeping it off will be an insurmountable challenge. Low fasting leptin levels mean that leptin is able to do its job and that your body won't sabotage your weight-loss efforts by making you constantly hungry.

More important, leptin levels are a bellwether as to how well a person is aging. If their leptin levels are high, it bodes ominously for their health, and that bodes poorly for longevity. In fact, remember those calorie-deprived laboratory animals that were much healthier and lived well beyond their normal life span that I described earlier? They had very low leptin levels compared to their well-fed peers. Fortunately, it is easy to lower your leptin levels without starvation by following the Rosedale Diet, as I'll describe later.

■ LEPTIN HELPS YOU LOSE FAT

When patients come to me saying that they would like to lose weight, what they are really saying is that they want to lose fat. No one wants to lose muscle or bone! The goal of dieting is to burn off excess fat so that it doesn't end up on your abdomen, thighs, rear end, or in your arteries where it can cause a heart attack. Leptin not only controls hunger, but it is the hormone that tells the body whether it should burn away excess fat. *This is one of the most critical messages that your body must hear to maintain normal weight and optimal health.*

When leptin levels can be properly "heard," it alerts your brain and other body tissues that you have eaten enough and stored away enough fat, and it's now time to burn off some excess fat. This feedback system is designed to prevent you from getting fat. In order for leptin to be heard clearly, however, leptin levels must remain stable and low. When leptin levels spike too high, too often, your cells stop listening to leptin. In medical terms, they become "resistant" to leptin's message. When your brain and other body tissues don't properly "hear" leptin's message, your brain continues to believe that you must hoard away even more fat for a rainy day. It tells you, "Be hungry, eat, and store more fat." Before too long, you will be fat.

If you want to lose weight, and keep it off, you must first maintain lower leptin levels so that your brain and body tissues can relearn how to listen to leptin. I often refer to my diet as a *leptin sensitizing* diet as opposed to a weight-loss diet. The fact is, you can't do one successfully without the other. When leptin sensitivity is restored, you will stop storing excess fat and instead, start burning it off. Best of all, your hunger will be controlled, you will not have food cravings, and you will have a trim, well-toned, and healthy body.

■ THE OPTIMAL DIET

Unlike stereotypical "dieters," my patients don't "yo-yo" up and down the scale, nor do they flit from my diet to the next fad diet. Most have stayed with me for years, and the reason they stay is that my diet works. The Rosedale Diet is dramatically different from standard weight loss diets, which I believe is the key to its success.

The average American has such poor eating habits that making any change is likely going to be an improvement, but that's not saying much.

Follow any of the popular weight-loss diets, and you'll probably lose some weight, but you won't be restoring leptin sensitivity as effectively, so you'll still be battling hunger. Moreover, simply losing weight does not necessarily mean that you are losing weight in a *healthy* way, or that you'll be able to keep it off. Eating for optimal health as well as to lose weight is a greater challenge, and doing it for the long-term is a greater challenge yet. Yet that is exactly what the Rosedale Diet does.

Virtually all of the popular diets today are basically variations on the same two themes: (1) the high carbohydrate–low fat diet (heavy in grains, starches, salads, and fruit) or (2) the high protein–low carbohydrate diet (heavy in meat, fish, poultry, dairy, and eggs). Neither type is as effective as mine, and no popular diet other than the Rosedale Diet has been shown to control leptin.

As its name implies, the high carbohydrate–low fat diet severely restricts fat intake. You can't eat much protein because it is often high in fat, and you are forced to eat mostly starches (like pasta), grains, and salads. As I will explain later, many carbohydrates—even the ones you think are healthy—can cause those spikes in leptin that will make you leptin-resistant.

The all-the-protein-you-can-eat-diet fixates on eating protein and ignores fat. Your plate is piled high with meat of any kind, and as much as you like, but you are severely restricted in your carbohydrate intake. The dirty secret of high protein diets is that if you eat more protein than your body requires, the excess can turn toxic and can threaten your health. There is even growing evidence that a high protein diet significantly increases your risk of heart disease, another fact you won't hear from proponents of these diets.

In contrast to the standard other weight-loss diets, *the Rosedale Diet focuses on fat—burning fat and eating fat.* In fact, it allows you to eat up to *half* or more of your daily calories in the form of fat, as long as it's the right kind of fat. Since fat is what gives food much of its flavor and texture, eating a high fat diet is hardly a hardship. You also eat protein on my diet, but in the right amount, because excessive protein consumption can be dangerous. You can also eat a fair amount of carbohydrate, but only the healthy ones that won't cause the precipitous spikes in leptin that are so damaging to health.

▪ FAT CAN BE GOOD

It may seem counterintuitive—even reckless—to recommend that overweight people eat more fat. Haven't we been told that fat is what makes you fat, and that fat is what causes heart disease? Actually, this is only half true. Eating fat does not necessarily make you fat and unhealthy . . . not being able to burn fat does. Furthermore, not all fat is the same. Fat can be your best friend or your worst enemy. Some fat is bad, notably excess amounts of most *saturated fat*, found in most meat and in full fat dairy products and omega-6 fats found in many kinds of vegetable oils. So, too, are trans fats found in fried and many processed foods. These "killer" fats can increase the risk of heart disease, diabetes, and a myriad of other health problems. That's one of the reasons why I don't like high protein and other low carb diets which do not distinguish between killer fats and good fats.

Trying to cut *all* fat out of our diets, we have eliminated the good fats: monounsaturated fats and omega-3 fatty acids. These fats are found in foods that are often restricted in other diets, but not on mine. On the Rosedale Diet, you can eat nuts such as almonds, walnuts, cashews and nut butters, avocados (yes, on my diet you can eat guacamole), fatty fish, non grain-fed beef, omega-3 enriched eggs, and high quality vegetable oils. Our bodies thrive on good fat. Our metabolism needs good fat to burn bad fat. Our cells need good fat to work properly. Our brains need good fat to think. Most important, good fat lowers leptin levels, improving the quality of leptin signaling so that our cells hear leptin better, thereby controlling hunger. *Remember, eating fat doesn't make you fat—the inability to burn fat is what makes you fat.* Good fat turns you into a wonderful fat burner. It is truly a miracle food.

▪ HOW I LEARNED ABOUT THE LEPTIN LINK

As founder of the North Carolina Center for Metabolic Medicine, cofounder of the Colorado Center for Metabolic Medicine, and founder of Rosedale Metabolic Medicine in Denver, Colorado, I have

GOOD-BYE FOOD CRAVINGS . . . HELLO TASTE BUDS

When your cells can't "hear" leptin's messages, you will not only be hungry all the time, but you will crave *sweets*. Why? Leptin resistance desensitizes your taste buds to sugar. That means, the more sugary foods you eat, the less likely you are to discern a sweet taste, so you will need more and more high-sugar snacks to feel satisfied. Whereas once almonds, blueberries or cinnamon tea would taste sweet enough to be treats, you now require multiple sugar hits—cookies, cake, candy bars, soft drinks, or a pint of ice cream—before you feel you've had enough. Once leptin sensitivity is restored and your taste buds shift into high gear, you will get much more pleasure from eating. You will rediscover the natural sweetness in food and will actually find that the supersweet snacks you once craved now taste sickeningly sweet.

treated patients from all over the world, many of whom are casualties of other diets. I attracted a great deal of attention in the medical community nine years ago when I was one of the first doctors to lecture about the importance of insulin resistance and by showing that I was able to cure, yes, *cure*, many cases of diabetes through diet alone.

As many of you know, there are two types of diabetes: type 1 and type 2. Type 1 diabetes (also called juvenile diabetes) is a result of too little insulin, the hormone that is produced in response to rising blood sugar levels. Without enough insulin, blood sugar levels can climb dangerously high, leading to organ damage and death. Type 2 diabetes (also called adult-onset diabetes) is an entirely different story. Type 2 diabetes is characterized by a condition called insulin resistance, which occurs when the cells of the body are constantly exposed to high levels of insulin. When you become insulin resistant, your body is making enough insulin, but your cells do not utilize it effectively. (The same thing occurs with leptin, causing leptin resistance.)

I lecture frequently to medical groups, and I am passionate about teaching other physicians that food is indeed the most powerful medicine. I believe that physicians should strive to get patients on a good diet and off drugs, whenever possible. It has become fashionable these days to quote Hippocrates, who said, "Let food be your medicine and medicine be your food." In my case, that philosophy is the cornerstone of my medical practice.

I am also a well-known specialist in the field of aging, and lecture on that topic as well. It is not unrelated to diabetes. In fact, my interest in diabetes was sparked by the observation that diabetics suffered from the so-called diseases of aging, such as arthritis, heart disease, cataracts, and even dementia at a much earlier age than normal. They even *look* older at an early age. From that realization, it dawned on me that the metabolic disorder of diabetes is a disease of rapid aging, and what we consider to be the "normal" diseases of aging are in reality due to an underlying disease of metabolic dysfunction.

I have come to believe that leptin resistance is at least related to, if not at the foundation of the majority of disorders related to aging, including heart disease, diabetes, obesity, osteoporosis, arthritis, and even aging itself. I know that many of you are probably thinking, how could one hormone—let alone a hormone that most of you have probably never even heard of before—be so important to health and longevity? In the chapters to come, I'll answer this question and you will see the critical role that leptin plays in your body.

Modern medicine has focused on merely treating symptoms, such as high cholesterol or elevated blood sugar, and not the true disease that underlies those symptoms, for that is far easier . . . and therefore more lucrative. My experience has taught me that treating symptoms simply masks problems, and will almost always make them worse, not better. If you lower leptin to healthy levels, you will go a long way toward preventing and treating a main root of what we call the diseases of aging and, in fact, aging itself. I believe that the diseases of aging are not inevitable, and that they are aggravated, if not caused, by the typically poor American diet.

■ DE-AGE YOUR BODY WITH THE ROSEDALE DIET

When I say that I believe in the power of food, I mean it. I have found that the Rosedale Diet is much more effective medicine than any combination of drugs and surgery could ever be. I don't write prescriptions for so-called longevity drugs like growth hormone or other "magic" anti-aging medicines. I don't prescribe drugs for weight loss, and am very against the use of any so-called thermogenic agents like ephedra (ma huang), which has been banned by the FDA, and caffeine to lose weight. They are not safe or particularly effective and, moreover, they actually can accelerate the aging process. I believe that proper diet is the primary way to achieve permanent weight loss, optimal health, and a longer life.

I also recommend nutritional supplements, but there is no supplement that can undo the damage of a poor diet. You need to eat well to make the supplements work well.

I am a metabolic specialist who has devoted my career to treating diseases such as obesity, heart disease, and diabetes. My interest in metabolism began when I was a medical student at Northwestern University, and I had the privilege of working with Dr. Jeremiah Stamler, one of the first to study the correlation between elevated cholesterol and heart disease. Until then, the medical establishment had all but ignored the role of diet in disease. It was already thought that a high fat diet could increase cholesterol levels in the body, and after his research, everyone jumped on the "no fat–no cholesterol" bandwagon. We were told that the ideal diet was low in fat and cholesterol, and high in carbohydrates, especially for diabetics, who were at greater risk of heart disease. We didn't know about leptin yet, nor did we understand the role of insulin in metabolic disease, nor did we differentiate between good fats and bad fats. I saw diabetic patients on this so-called ideal diet get worse, not better. Worst of all, they were always hungry and couldn't stay on that diet. I asked myself why the standard diet wasn't working. If fat was the culprit, why were diabetic patients on the low fat diet getting worse and developing high triglycerides and other lipid abnormalities? Why did most of them require more, not less medicine on this diet? Why were they so unhappy and so hungry?

One day it dawned on me that the high carbohydrate–low fat diet that was being prescribed to diabetic patients was precisely the wrong therapeutic approach. The reason why now seems obvious, but a decade ago, it was revolutionary bordering on heretical. Carbohydrate in any form other than fiber is eventually metabolized by the body into sugar. In fact, it starts turning into sugar as soon as it hits the saliva in your mouth. It doesn't matter if it's a piece of fruit, a brownie, or a bowl of whole grain cereal, it still turns to sugar, and feeding sugar to a diabetic to lower blood sugar is nonsensical. (There are some carbs that are better for you than others, but nevertheless, any carb that is not fiber eventually ends up as sugar.)

■ EXCESS PROTEIN IS JUST AS BAD

If high carbohydrate wasn't the right approach, that left two other major food categories on which to base a diet: protein and fat. It may surprise you to learn that the protein that the body doesn't quickly use to repair or make new cells is largely broken down into simple sugars, which increases blood sugar and promotes insulin resistance. Furthermore, protein itself triggers insulin production, which can worsen insulin resistance. (That is why diabetics should never go on a very high protein diet.)

Having ruled out carbohydrates and protein, I decided to try putting my diabetic patients on a high fat diet, but only using healthy fats, such as those you'll eat on the Rosedale Diet. When I switched my patients to this new diet, I saw vast improvements in nearly every case. In addition to losing a lot of unwanted weight, patients were able to reduce or eliminate their medication. And they never complained that they were hungry. I was so impressed with these results that I recommended the diet for my nondiabetic patients who were trying to lose weight, many of whom were insulin resistant. The weight literally melted off them, and most were able to keep it off. Years later, after the discovery of leptin, I found out why my diet worked so well. It lowered leptin levels quickly and effectively. I also discovered why the other diets had failed. They didn't lower leptin levels nearly as well or as effectively; in fact, they often raised leptin levels! (Shockingly, most diabetics are still being treated with the high carbohydrate–low fat diet.) I offer the only alternative that works, and works fabulously well and works the best: the Rosedale Diet.

■ "LISTENING" TO LEPTIN

When leptin was first discovered in 1995, it was dubbed the "holy grail of weight loss," and there were high hopes among the scientific community that the cure for obesity had finally been found. Initially, scientists believed that if you gave overweight people supplementary leptin, it would stimulate fat burning. But when they measured leptin levels in overweight people, they were in for a big surprise. Most overweight people—and nearly all obese people—are not leptin deficient; in fact, they produce *too much leptin*. As a result, they become leptin resistant, much the same the way people with type 2 diabetes are insulin resistant.

When a person becomes leptin resistant, it takes more and more leptin to tell the brain that it's satisfied and that you don't need more food. Therefore, it takes more and more food to feel satisfied. The brain, not hearing leptin, frantically signals for more and more fat to be stored. Since leptin is made by fat cells, you have to make more and more fat to produce enough leptin to finally get its message across to the brain to stop being hungry and stop storing fat. This creates a vicious cycle: you eat more because your brain doesn't know how to tell you to stop, and the only way you can stop is by producing more fat to make more leptin, which means that you keep getting fatter, and more insulin and leptin resistant, which just makes you want to keep eating more.

Certain foods feed into this vicious cycle by triggering a huge surge in leptin production. Carbohydrates—including breads, grains, cereals, pastas, and starchy vegetables—are the worst offenders. When you eat these foods, your leptin levels soar. These foods can create even more mischief because they are broken down into simple sugars that can be rapidly burned by the body. If sugar is available, and your body is given a choice between burning fat and burning sugar, it burns mostly sugar. So all that fat you have socked away stays exactly where it is. Here's the kicker. What happens to extra sugar that isn't burned? It gets made into saturated fat, which is resistant to burning. What happens to all that stored extra fat? It produces even more leptin in response to sugar, which worsens leptin resistance.

Are high protein diets any better? Protein is used to repair and rejuvenate the body, but the body can only use a limited amount of protein at a time. What isn't used is largely converted into glucose (a form of sugar), and burned. What isn't burned is made into fat—saturated fat. To compound the problem, most of the protein we eat today, particularly beef and chicken, are grain-fed to fatten them up, not just grass-fed as they were in the old days. Grain feeding produces animals much higher in saturated fat than normal. I often refer to the fat in grain-fed animals as "second generation starch," because the starchy carbohydrates that the animals eat will ultimately be stored as fat in us. Thus, the longtime nutritional advice of the medical profession to eat a high carbohydrate, low saturated fat diet is an oxymoron!

The First Step—Lower Leptin

From my experience with thousands of patients I have learned that once you *lower* leptin levels and regain leptin sensitivity, leptin can then begin to do its vital job of turning off the hunger switch and turning on the fat-burning switch. Any weight-loss diet that does not lower leptin quickly is putting the cart before the horse and will ultimately fail.

On the Rosedale Diet, fasting leptin levels are greatly reduced long before you see any appreciable weight loss. People are allowed to eat whenever they are hungry, and as frequently as they would like. If they're eating fewer calories, it is only because they are not hungry due to improved leptin sensitivity. That is why people are able to follow my diet so successfully.

Good Fat Lowers Leptin

It is a well-known fact that 90 percent of all dieters quickly regain the weight they lost after dieting. I'm not surprised and I can't say that I blame them. The fact is, if you don't solve the leptin problem, you won't solve the hunger problem, and if you don't turn off the hunger switch, almost anyone will eventually give in and eat. There is only one diet that lowers leptin quickly and effectively—a diet that contains adequate amounts of GOOD FAT and is low in starch and sugar—the Rosedale Diet.

So, what is good fat?

- Good fat does not stimulate a surge in leptin production—rather it suppresses it.
- Good fat is not burned as sugar like carbohydrates and protein—it is burned as fat.
- Good fat stimulates the body to burn more fat.

What happens when we don't eat enough good fat? Paradoxically, we become fat because we can't burn off excess fat.

■ LIVE LONGER: BECOME A FAT BURNER

Every time you eat, you are feeding the trillions of cells throughout the body. Our cells need fuel to repair and regenerate themselves, and to do the body's work. Our cells can eat two kinds of food—sugar or fat. Unfortunately, as we get older, our bodies become accustomed to burning the one particular fuel used most often—sugar—and are less flexible about burning the other fuel—fat.

Most people are good sugar burners because they've had a lot of experience doing so, due to our typically high sugar and starch diet. Even when you are not eating, your body's cells are still burning fuel to do their work. When you are a sugar burner, your body continues to burn sugar as its primary fuel and to sock away fat. I call this phenomenon "metabolic momentum." The body continues to burn the fuel it is accustomed to burning. Being essentially a 24/7 sugar burner can be very damaging. Your body can't store very much sugar. To continue to feed its sugar habit when you don't eat, your body will break down the protein in its lean tissues—including muscle and bone—into sugar. Your body would prefer not to destroy itself in this way, so it will make you hungry and make you crave sugar. This makes you more and more leptin resistant. And instead of burning off excess fat, you make more of it, and you store more of it away. Over time you end up turning your muscle and bone into sugar and fat as you get fatter, weaker, more frail, and flabbier. And you will always be hungry.

If you eat sugar (or foods that turn into sugar) and fat together, the body will burn the sugar and store the fat. Sugar and fat is a common combination—think of buttered toast! Our cells are hardwired to burn sugar first: no one knows why this is so, but there are probably good reasons for this. Excess sugar poses a far greater threat to your body than excess fat (which isn't good either, but is not quite as bad as sugar—diabetes can kill you faster!). When sugar combines with the proteins in your body (called glycation), it triggers chemical reactions that can be very damaging to healthy cells and can cause aging, disease, and death. Sugar burning also promotes the formation of potentially high amounts of toxic chemicals called free radicals, unstable oxygen molecules that can damage cells and ultimately lead to numerous diseases. My hunch is, the body probably burns off sugar first as a defense mechanism to protect you from the potentially lethal effects of sugar. Thus, if we bombard our bodies with sugar-producing foods, it becomes harder for our bodies to switch to fat-burning mode.

Being a chronic sugar burner can have serious health consequences, but the primary one is that it causes weight gain (because you rarely burn up your fat) which can cause serious health problems, including insulin resistance. Being a sugar burner will also age you faster, and can shorten your life, as I will explain in Chapter 4. By eating good fat, we can retrain our bodies to become fat burners. Being a fat burner has its advantages—once your cells begin to burn off fat for fuel, metabolic momentum takes over. Even when you don't eat, your cells will continue to keep burning stored fat, making you feel am often asked to briefly summarize what it is that establishes health. I can do this in a single sentence. "Health and life span is determined by the proportion of fat versus sugar people burn throughout their lifetime" The more fat you burn as fuel, the healthier you will be. The more sugar you burn as fuel, the more disease-ridden you will be, and the shorter your life will likely be.

more satisfied and less hungry. Needless to say, when you're not carrying around all that excess fat, you'll be trimmer, more attractive, and healthier.

How Do You Become a Champion Fat Burner?

As the saying goes, practice makes perfect. The only way you get good at something is by doing it frequently. You can become a good tennis player by playing tennis and you become a good golfer by playing golf. You become a good fat burner by burning fat. To do so you must limit your sugar and foods that turn into sugar (including starch and excess protein), especially for the first few weeks when your metabolism is learning to switch from burning sugar to burning fat. You need to break the negative "metabolic momentum" that is locking you into toxic fat storage–sugar burning mode, and locking you out of fat burning.

■ KNOW YOUR LEPTIN LEVELS

Although I recommend that everyone have their leptin levels checked as part of their routine annual physical, you can still benefit from the Rosedale Diet if you don't. Whether or not you know your precise leptin levels, as you slim down, you will be "losing leptin" along with excess fat.

What is a healthy leptin level? When you have leptin levels

checked, your doctor sends a sample of your blood (after an overnight fast) to a laboratory for analysis where you will be given a numerical rating. Many, but not all laboratories do leptin analysis. In Chapter 10, "The Leptin Test and Other Medical Tests That Can Save Your Life," I provide a list of laboratories that check leptin, and will explain what the test results mean.

Most obese people have very elevated leptin levels. Within two to three weeks on the Rosedale Diet, nearly everyone will experience a dramatic decline in leptin levels. I often retest my patients at this point to see how they are doing. At the same time, you will find that you do not get hungry as often as you used to, that you no longer experience the food cravings that you used to, and that you will have little difficulty following the diet. Younger people have quicker results than older people, who often have more damage to undo. In some cases, leptin levels do not fall as quickly as they should. To me it's a sign that those people need to be extra careful about sticking to the diet, and that they may need additional support, including extra nutritional supplements.

■ LIVE LONGER, LIVE STRONGER

There's yet another advantage the Rosedale Diet has over other diets. Unlike other diets, where you lose muscle along with fat, on my diet, *you lose only fat and excess fluid,* so you don't look thin and flabby; you look as good as you feel. There is a good scientific reason why this happens. Once leptin sensitivity is restored, your cells also become sensitized to other hormones such as insulin and IGF-1, which are instrumental in muscle development. If your hormonal signaling is out of whack, you can diet forever and exercise until you drop, but you will still not be able to burn off fat and get lean. Once your cells begin "hearing" the correct hormonal signals, they do their jobs better and faster. Countless patients have told me that once they've started following the Rosedale Diet they're working out less, but making more progress.

I recommend that you do some exercise on my program, but you only need to do a small amount—about fifteen minutes of mild exercise daily. To me, exercise is the "gravy" of the Rosedale Diet. A little exercise goes a long way as long as you're following the good plan.

■ HOW THE DIET WORKS

The Rosedale Diet is divided into two levels. Everyone follows Level 1 for the first three weeks of the program. I view the first twenty-one days as a training period in which you teach your metabolism to burn fat instead of sugar. During this time, you will eat foods that are high in good fat, and virtually no starchy or sugary carbohydrates. You will, however, be allowed to load up on all the high-fiber vegetables you want. It's a very healthy and satisfying way to eat. Some of you should continue to follow Level 1 forever, particularly those of you with metabolic disorders such as diabetes or coronary artery disease, or those of you who want to stave off the aging process for as long as possible. Most people find it much easier than they originally thought it would be after having been on it, and after having changed their metabolic chemistry. It is the ideal way to eat. If, however, you do not have a health problem, you can move on to Level 2, which does contain somewhat more starch and sugar, although only the healthiest kind with the highest fiber content. (No candy bars, please!)

■ FOOD FOR LIFE

I'm often asked, "Once I lose all the weight I want, do I need to stay on the diet?" I consider the Rosedale Diet the optimal diet for life and I urge patients to stay on it forever. If you keep your leptin levels down, you will not experience the constant hunger or food cravings that helped make you overweight and sick in the first place, and that makes diets difficult or impossible to maintain! After you achieve your desired weight (once you become a good fat burner), some of you may be able to eat more starchy carbohydrates than I recommend (in the more liberal Level 2 plan) and not have any problems. You can indulge in an extra serving of bread a day or an occasional plate of pasta, and still keep the weight off, if you stick to the program for most other meals. Once you become a good fat burner, you can also eat a little more saturated fat. The kind of fat you eat becomes less important because you are able to burn it off more easily.

Many people, however, cannot deviate from the program. Once they fall off the diet, they become leptin resistant once again and begin to experience food cravings and rapid weight gain. They quickly lose their ability to be fat burners and begin hoarding fat. If you have a history of food cravings and overeating, it is imperative that you simply stay on the diet. If you go off the diet and begin to experience weight gain, go right back on it.

Once you've slimmed down and regained your leptin sensitivity, if you do indulge in an occasional high-starch, high-carbohydrate meal, you can burn it off by doing exercise after eating. Fifteen minutes of vigorous exercise can burn up the sugar. Once you are no longer leptin resistant, your body's hormonal signaling will be able to bounce back to normal more quickly. If, however, you go back to your old eating habits, you will quickly become leptin resistant, and this quick exercise fix won't work.

■ HOW TO USE THIS BOOK

The Rosedale Diet is divided into three parts:

Part I, "Everything You Need to Know About the Rosedale Diet," contains all the information you need to understand the solid science behind the Rosedale Diet, and why leptin is key to your health.

Part II, "Making the Rosedale Diet Work for You," is divided into seven sections: "Why Good Fat Does a Body Good," "The Rosedale Diet Guide to Healthy Eating," "Getting Started: Weeks One to Three," "A Guide to the Rosedale Diet Supplement Program," "Rosedale Diet Exercise Strategies," "The Leptin Test and Other Medical Tests That Can Save Your Life," and "Getting Healthy with the Rosedale Diet," which provides information on the treatment of leptin-related disorders, including diabetes, heart disease, osteoporosis and arthritis.

"Rosedale Resources" provides original recipes and other vital information that will help incorporate the Rosedale Diet into your life.

■ COMMONLY ASKED QUESTIONS ABOUT
THE ROSEDALE DIET

I think that I'm a nervous eater. I eat even when I'm not hungry. How can your program help me?

The Rosedale Diet is perfect for people who categorize themselves as "nervous eaters." As I explain in Chapters 3 and 4, elevated levels of leptin actually stimulate the production of stress hormones, which can make you very jittery. Lowering leptin levels and restoring leptin sensitivity will have a calming effect on your body and your mind. Second, your feelings of nervousness may actually be symptoms of food "withdrawal" due to malfunctioning hunger signals to your brain. When leptin sensitivity is restored and your brain can "listen" to leptin, you will know when you are truly hungry, and you will not experience "false hunger" or feel compelled to eat when you don't need to.

I heard that high protein diets are dangerous because they cause ketosis. Does a high fat diet cause similar problems?

First of all, let me correct a popular misconception about high protein diets and ketones. Ketones are a by-product of fat burning, and they are a good, efficient fuel. Under normal circumstances, your cells should be able to burn ketones and keep them at a low level. It is healthy for cells to burn ketones, especially your brain cells. In fact, the so-called ketogenic diet is now the treatment of choice for epilepsy where drug therapy has failed.

Ketosis is often confused with ketoacidosis, which occurs in severe uncontrolled diabetes when virtually no insulin is produced and ketones are allowed to build up to extraordinarily high levels, which can be dangerous. This is not to say that I think a high protein diet is good; it's bad for other reasons. Protein is acidic and is broken down into two potentially toxic waste products: urea and ammonia. You don't want to overload your body with these nasty by-products of protein metabolism.

Furthermore, the more protein you eat, the more proficient you become at making glucose from the protein in your diet, and from the protein in your muscle and bone. As I tell my diabetic patients, this is something that you don't want to be good at! Remember, you need to eat enough protein to replace and repair body parts, but not so much that you must burn off the excess as sugar, thus disrupting your metabolism. On the other hand, a high fat diet is best as long as you eat primarily good fats, and don't eat sugar-forming foods with it.

Does daily calorie intake matter?

I don't ask people to count calories because I believe that counting calories as a diet tool doesn't work. For years, people have been told that cutting back on calories is the way to lose weight and keep it off. The result of this poor advice is yo-yo dieting and the obesity epidemic we have today. Calories do matter, but you cannot diet for very long by using willpower and simply relying on your ability to eat less food despite hunger. Hunger is an extremely powerful, ancient urge and it's unrealistic to expect people to walk around hungry when they don't have to. You can only reduce calories long-term by not *wanting* to eat. That means not being hungry. Most people actually do eat fewer calories on the Rosedale Diet than they did, but not because I force them to. They eat less because they are satiated more easily, and do not desire more food.

You want people to eat more good fat. How do I know how much fat I'm eating every day? Should I count fat grams?

The Rosedale Diet will correct the hormonal signals that tell you how much to eat and how to access fat that you have been storing in your belly's cupboard for years so that your cells can eat fat without your having to. Remember, it is your cells that eat, and I want them to be burning fat almost all of the time. Some diets require that you count the number of fat grams that you consume each day. I think it's a waste of your time. The Rosedale Diet sample menus will give you a good idea of how to incorporate foods containing the right amount of good fat into your daily diet. If you follow the program, you will get the right amount of the right kind of fat. Is there a chance that some of you will gorge on fat? I don't think so. When your cells become leptin sensitive once again, you are much less likely to overeat, and much more likely to eat normal portion sizes.

I don't like fish. Can I still follow your program?

Absolutely! You are required to eat a certain amount of protein every day, and preferably protein that contains good fat, but it doesn't have to come from fish. If you review the food lists on pages 103–117, you will see that there is a wide variety of foods from which you can plan your meals. I also recommend that everyone take a fish oil supplement daily (I know what you're thinking: Yuck! In fact, the fish oil supplement that I recommend actually tastes fine, and is acceptable even to most fish haters. See page 149.)

I'm not overweight; can I still benefit from your program?

The Rosedale Diet is a diet designed to achieve optimal mental and physical health, and to extend both your life span and your health span. Your ability to burn fat is key to determining how healthy you are and how long you will live. Many of my patients do not need to lose weight, but are interested in living as long a life as possible, and as healthy a life as possible. I believe that the Rosedale Diet will help them achieve both those goals.

Are you leptin resistant? Take the quiz in Chapter 2 to see whether you have any of the warning signs or symptoms of leptin resistance, and how they can undermine your weight loss efforts and your health.

chapter two

Are You Leptin Resistant? Take This Quiz

H ow do you know if you are leptin resistant? You can know for sure by having your leptin levels checked by your doctor (see Chapter 10). There are also some telltale signs of leptin resistance, which I describe below. Please take the following test to see if you have any warning signs of leptin resistance, and why those signs are significant.

1. *When you go on a weight loss diet, do you have trouble losing fat, that is, do you lose pounds but still remain flabby?*

Yes _____ No _____

What This Symptom Means. If you are leptin resistant, it is a sign that you are eating a diet that promotes the production and storage of fat, and the burning of sugar as your body's primary fuel. Ideally, you want to retool your body's metabolic machinery so that you burn fat as your primary fuel. You're not going to become a fat burner simply by cutting back on calories, following a high carbohydrate–low fat diet, or going on a high protein diet. The only way to retool your metabolic machinery is to eat a diet that is rich in good fat, contains the right amount of protein, and is very low in starchy and sugary carbohydrates. What happens if you go on a weight loss diet, but are still burning sugar as your primary fuel? Ultimately, you will lose muscle. Why? In the absence of sugar from your food, your body will burn protein from your lean mass for fuel, and you will lose muscle. At the end of all your dieting, you will still be flabby, and you will still be burning sugar and hoarding fat. Remember, it isn't weight you want to lose—it's *fat*—and the only way you can lose fat is by becoming a fat burner.

2. *Do you have trouble keeping weight off after dieting?*

Yes _____ No _____

What This Symptom Means. Most people can take weight off fairly quickly, but keeping it off is the real challenge. If you simply take off weight, but do not restore leptin sensitivity, you will have an extremely difficult time maintaining your weight loss. If your cells can't "hear" leptin's cues, you will feel hungry even when your body doesn't need food, and your body will think it should be storing fat when in fact it should be burning fat. You may even get fatter while trying to eat less because your body will try even harder to hold on to fat as you cut back on food.

3. *Are you constantly hungry?*

Yes _____ No _____

What This Symptom Means. Is your stomach always growling for food? Constant hunger is one of the *early* signs of leptin resistance. If you find that you are suddenly getting hungry at odd times during the day (or night) and are eating more, your leptin signaling is off. When things are going right, leptin lets your brain know that your cells have enough fuel to do their work, and blocks the urge to eat.

4. *Do you crave sweets?*

Yes _____ No _____

What This Symptom Means. As noted in Chapter 1, leptin resistance actually desensitizes your taste buds to sugar, so you need to eat more and more sweets to feel satisfied. Ironically, as you eat more and more sweets, you actually enjoy them less. Yet you find them impossible to resist. This leads to destructive binge eating and unwanted weight gain.

5. *Do you wake up hungry at night?*

Yes _____ No _____

What This Symptom Means. Nights are for sleeping, not for eating. Sleep is a time when your body is supposed to take a break from the stress of digestion so it can wind down and concentrate on (1) maintenance and repair of your cells to keep you in peak condition and, in the process (2) burn up fat stores as fuel to do this repair work. If you're hungry at night, it is usually because you have run out of sugar to burn and your body has "forgotten" how to burn fat. The fact is, you should be able to get adequate nourishment during the day and burn fat stores at night so that you don't feel hungry at night. If your leptin signaling is off, however, you will feel hungry when you shouldn't, even when you should be sleeping.

6. *Do you have a "spare tire" or an apple shape?*

Yes _____ No _____

What This Symptom Means. When you are leptin resistant your body not only makes too much fat, it loses the knowledge of where to put all that fat. Fat can be stored in two major depots; under your skin (known as subcutaneous fat) or around your internal organs (known as visceral fat or midline obesity). Leptin resistance causes fat to accumulate around your "middle," which leads to an apple-shaped body. Midline obesity is associated with a much higher risk of multiple diseases, including heart disease and diabetes.

7. *Are you losing muscle mass despite the fact that you are exercising?*

Yes _____ No _____

What This Symptom Means. If you are leptin resistant, you can work out until you are blue in the face, but your body will still be programmed to chew up muscle and store fat. You will not be getting anywhere close to the full benefit of your workout. When it comes to maintaining lean body mass, eating the right diet is even more critical than working out. If you are a sugar burner/fat storer, your body will continue to burn lean mass as sugar even when you are not eating and you will be working harder and harder to keep whatever muscle you have. When your cells regain their hormonal sensitivity, it will take a lot less exercise to maintain your muscle.

8. *Do you feel stressed out?*

Yes _____ No _____

What This Symptom Means. Leptin resistance stimulates the production of stress hormones, which keep your body revved up and you feeling anxious and stressed-out. Many people respond to stress by overeating, reaching for so-called comfort foods—sugary and starchy carbohydrates. This will only aggravate leptin resistance, and make you more stressed-out and fatter (and stressed-out about being fat).

9. *Have you been diagnosed with high triglyceride levels?*

Yes _____ No _____

What This Symptom Means. Triglycerides are a fancy medical name for fat. Your blood level of triglycerides is a measure of the amount of fat floating around your bloodstream. If your triglycerides are high, you are either making too much fat or burning too little. Elevated triglycerides are associated with an increased risk of heart attack and stroke. (I recommend that everyone have their triglycerides checked at their annual physical examination. See page 177.) Elevated triglycerides are very common among overweight and obese people, and are typically a direct result of eating a high carbohydrate–low fat diet. If you are leptin resistant, you are making and storing excess fat and not burning it, and therefore are vulnerable to having elevated triglycerides.

10. *Do you have high blood pressure?*

Yes _____ No_____

What This Symptom Means. Leptin resistance can cause hormonal changes that trigger the production of stress hormones, which can raise blood pressure. It also causes excess fluid to accumulate, contributing to high blood pressure. High blood pressure is very common among people with midline "abdominal" obesity, insulin resistance, high triglycerides, and who are overweight.

11. *Have you been diagnosed with osteoporosis?*

Yes _____ No_____

What This Symptom Means. I bet you're surprised to see this question here, but leptin resistance puts you at great risk of osteoporosis, the potentially debilitating disease characterized by the thinning of bone. It's important to remember that your cells are eating even when you are not. Your body continues to burn fuel to do the work of maintaining life long after you have stopped eating, even when you are sleeping. If your body is used to burning sugar, it will continue to burn sugar. Your body can't store too much sugar away at one time—instead, it converts extra sugar and stores it as fat. So what's a body to do when it prefers to eat sugar, but it has already burned up what you ate at your last meal? It will look for sugar from other sources, and the protein in muscle and bone is the ultimate source. Moreover, high levels of leptin actually inhibit the ability of special cells called osteoblasts to make new bone. If you want to prevent osteoporosis, the first and most important step is to restore leptin sensitivity so that you can stop burning sugar and breaking down your lean mass and start making new bone. (Please see page 192 for more information on osteoporosis.)

If you answered "yes" to any of these questions, you are likely to be suffering the symptoms of leptin resistance, and the devastating effects of being a sugar burner as opposed to being a fat burner. If you are leptin resistant, your metabolism is malfunctioning and your health will be seriously compromised. In Chapter 3, The Vicious Cycle, I explain why leptin resistance is so dangerous, and why it is so important not to ignore these telltale symptoms.

■ IN HER OWN WORDS ■

J. H., AGE 47

"When I was heavy, the first thing that I would do when I walked into a room was look around and see if I was the largest person there. That's not a healthy way to think!"

When I first starting seeing Ron, I weighed 173 pounds and I'm only 5'2"! I now weigh 122 pounds, and it has dramatically changed my outlook on life. I went to see Ron for two reasons. First, I was unhappy about my weight and how I looked, but I was also worried about my health. My dad had developed type 2 diabetes and I could see the terrible effect diabetes was having on his life, and I did not want to follow in his footsteps. I knew that if I kept gaining weight, I would probably become diabetic myself.

Over the years, I had been on many diets, primarily low fat, high carb diets, and while I would lose weight initially, I would put the weight right back on when I started eating normally again. These diets were very hard to stay on, and I would go on and off them. I actually bought a book about the Atkins diet, but the first two weeks on the diet (the induction period) looked so awful, I couldn't bring myself to do it. Once I started on Ron's program, it was pretty easy to follow. It's really a mindset. You have to decide that you are going to change the way you eat. The most remarkable thing is that I don't feel hungry all the time anymore, and when I do feel hungry, I eat. I grab a handful of nuts, I'm fine.

What's been the biggest change in my life since losing all that weight? My self-esteem has vastly improved. When I was heavy, the first thing that I would do when I walked into a room was look around and see if I was the largest person there. That's not a healthy way to think! I used to hate to go shopping. I had clothes in my closet from size 18 to size 8; I'm now a size 6. I feel really good about myself now.

chapter three

The Vicious Cycle: From Fat to Fatter

Are you putting on unwanted pounds with each passing year, and finding it harder and harder to take them off? Are you starting to dread your annual physical because your doctor is admonishing you to, "Get rid of that spare tire," "Lose some weight!" or "Watch your blood pressure!" Have you been diagnosed with heart disease, insulin resistance, or type 2 diabetes, or are you worried about a loved one who has?

If you're like most Americans, you're going to answer yes to at least one of these questions. The sad truth is, more than half of us are overweight, and a significant number of us are sick because of it. Here are the dismal statistics.

- The rate of obesity rose by 30 percent in the past ten years. One-third of all Americans are *obese*, meaning that they are so fat that their health is at serious risk.
- The incidence of type 2 diabetes (a disease that goes hand in hand with obesity) has tripled in the past 30 years, and is still heading upward. If present trends continue, that number will soar to 40 million by 2050.

- According to the Centers for Disease Control in Atlanta, 1 out of 3 children born in 2000 is destined to become diabetic unless there is a change in diet and lifestyle. That means that by mid twenty-first century, *one-third* of the adult population will be diabetic.
- Diabetes increases the risk of heart disease, kidney failure, cancer and dementia, which means that children born today will be at greater risk of these diseases as well.
- Obesity and overweight drain the U.S. health care system of more than $90 billion a year. Within a few decades, we could be spending double or even triple the amount on these diseases.

Most experts blame Americans for their own predicament, contending that we're getting sick and fat because we're eating too much and exercising too little. They offer overly simplistic solutions such as "just eat a little less" as the panacea to cure these vast health problems. As someone who understands the root cause of obesity, I can tell you that this is meaningless advice to give people who are leptin resistant, and that's the overwhelming majority of overweight and obese people. The primary message getting through to them is the one from their brain screaming, "Be hungry, eat, make more fat!" when that's the last thing they need to do. Unless you turn off this destructive message, you cannot treat obesity.

As a physician who has treated obesity and diabetes for decades with great success, I can tell you that the "just eat a little less" approach has done more harm than good. It is a classic example of how medicine fixates on the symptom but ignores the root cause. Certainly overeating combined with a sedentary lifestyle are contributing factors to obesity—but *why* is this happening in the first place? Why are people so out of control when it comes to their eating habits? Why do so many people suddenly have "supersized" appetites? What's happened in the past few decades that has rapidly accelerated the obesity epidemic?

Americans did not get into this mess because they lacked willpower, were natural gluttons, or were lazy. Moreover, solutions based on the "just eat a little less each day" further lock people into the vicious cycle that will ultimately leave them even fatter and sicker.

■ THE DESPERATE STRUGGLE

Americans may be getting fatter, but it's not for their lack of trying to slim down. Many of my patients have desperately tried to lose weight on their own, bouncing from one weight loss diet to the next. Many have joined gyms and have tried to become more physically active, but they have not been able to make a dent in either their obesity or their diabetes. In fact, most have gone from bad to worse following the standard "eat less and exercise more" advice. *It is almost impossible to eat less when there is a little devil on your shoulders born from leptin resistance that is constantly whispering to you, "eat more, get fatter."*

Numerous studies have documented that weight loss diets almost always fail, and that it is a rare person who is able to diet and keep the weight off. More often than not, within a year, dieters wind up even heavier than they were before they began the weight loss program. In fact, if you look at the fine print on television commercials or advertisements for diets in which successful dieters are trotted out to talk about the newest weight loss craze, you will always see a disclaimer noting that these good results are "atypical."

I can tell you with confidence that my good results are typical. My patients typically lose weight, keep it off, and regain their health. Why do my patients fare so well despite the abysmal odds against them? My approach to treating obesity is completely different from the standard approach. I don't consider obesity to be a disease; for that matter, I don't think of diabetes or heart disease as diseases. These conditions are symptoms of a greater underlying problem—the inability of the body to use energy correctly to maintain health and life. Instead of burning off extra fat, as our bodies were meant to do, the body hoards it. Going on a standard low calorie diet will just aggravate it. If we don't treat the underlying cause of this metabolic glitch, we will never truly cure obesity or diabetes—or any of the symptoms that we call disease, such as heart disease or osteoporosis—that feed on this vicious cycle. The underlying cause of the so-called diseases of aging is always a derangement in the cellular signals, the instructions that tell your body how to turn energy into life.

■ IT BEGINS IN THE WOMB

When does the vicious cycle begin? It may shock you to learn that it may begin as early as in the womb, before you are even born. If an expectant mother eats the wrong diet—that is, one deficient in good fat and loaded with high sugar carbohydrates—she could be passing on metabolic problems to her children, making them more vulnerable to becoming diabetic. The sad truth is that she is probably eating the diet recommended to her by her doctor! Animal studies have shown that insulin resistance, a precursor of type 2 diabetes, can be passed from an expectant mother to her child, and even worse, can alter the insulin sensitivity of the baby's eggs, thus possibly affecting the developing baby, and could affect that baby's children as well.

If you are insulin resistant, you are almost always leptin resistant, and if you are leptin resistant, you are a sugar burner, not a fat burner. If you are not burning fat, you are storing fat and getting fat. Is there any wonder why so many children today are overweight and obese? As of yet, there have not been any studies showing whether or not leptin resistance can be passed on this way, but there are clues that this is also true.

Whether or not you may be born with a tendency to develop leptin and insulin resistance, your diet is the primary force that will determine your destiny. If you eat the right food, your tendencies will stay suppressed. If you eat the wrong food, you will grow into an overweight, sick child or adult. Sadly, most kids are fed a diet almost opposite to what I recommend. From an early age, kids are put on a high carbohydrate diet, heavy in cereal, pasta, crackers, potatoes and fruit desserts. This sugar-loaded feast is then washed down with gallons of fruit juice. The diet I just described is not what is considered "junk food"; in fact, most parents and medical professions would consider it to be a wholesome diet. Why?

Because it doesn't contain a lot of fat! Many of you were probably raised on this type of diet yourself, and eat a similar diet today.

The "fat phobia" has created a mind-set in the medical community that borders on insanity. For example, I recently saw a box of chocolate-flavored breakfast cereal proudly displaying a stamp of approval from the American Heart Association. I was stunned. How could the American Heart Association approve of a breakfast cereal containing a whopping 26 grams of carbohydrate and 14 grams of added sugar! The cereal in question met their guidelines for being low in saturated fat. What the unsuspecting consumer doesn't know is that excess sugar is simply stored as saturated fat in the body, and if you regularly ate this cereal, I guarantee you would become leptin resistant and would eventually get fat.

What's wrong with the standard, high carbohydrate–low fat diet? As we explained in Chapters 1 and 2, your body runs best when it can burn fat. When you bombard your body with sugar via a high carbohydrate diet, it will almost exclusively burn sugar and store fat. You will become a proficient sugar burner and a poor fat burner. The end result is obesity and disease. *Remember, eating fat is not what makes you fat, it's the inability to burn fat that makes you fat.*

■ FROM BAD TO WORSE

In Chapter 1, I described how all carbohydrate (except for fiber) is broken down into sugar in the body. Starchy, sugary carbohydrates produce a rapid spike in leptin levels, the hormone produced by your fat cells. As you may remember, leptin should tell the brain that you have enough fat stored in your body, that you should stop making more fat, and that it's okay to start burning some off. It also lets your brain know when you have had enough food, and blocks the urge to eat.

Constant spikes in leptin levels throughout the day can cause a breakdown in communication between leptin and your cells. It's like having someone constantly yelling in your ear—eventually, you're going to protect yourself by getting earplugs to reduce the noise or you'll go deaf. Similarly, if your cells are constantly exposed to frequent spikes in leptin, they will stop listening. Over time, cells become desensitized to leptin, or leptin resistant. In order to get their message heard by the brain, fat cells have to produce more and more leptin so that they can "yell" louder and louder. This requires more and more fat to be made and stored. Because your brain has become "hard of hearing" to leptin there are no brakes on your appetite; you get hungrier and hungrier, eat more and more, get fatter and fatter, produce more and more leptin. . . . You get the idea. You get stuck in a most vicious of cycles. To further compound the problem, when your body is being told to make more and more fat, you won't burn it off, and you'll be forced to burn sugar. This triggers carbohydrate cravings to supply all that sugar, leading to more and more carbohydrate consumption, leptin spikes, and leptin resistance. Finally, as I mentioned earlier, studies show that excess leptin can interfere with the ability of your taste buds to taste sweets, so in order to experience a sweet flavor, you may have to eat more and more sugar, continuing your body's sugar burning pattern. You are burning sugar, storing fat, and getting fat. Even Superman would have trouble resisting the hormonal urges forcing you to eat and eat and eat.

▪ A MODERN EPIDEMIC

Leptin resistance is a relatively new phenomenon, aggravated by very recent changes in the modern diet. We have followed the medical profession's advice to eat less fat and to eat more carbohydrate. The food industry reaps the greatest profits from starchy carbohydrates (pasta, bread, cereals), which require far less money to preserve than foods high in fat, such as meat and fish, which require refrigeration during transport and in grocery stores.

The problem is, the human body was never meant to use sugar as its primary fuel: Sugar is the body's turbo charger fuel, the fuel you are supposed to use mostly when you need a sudden burst of energy. You've undoubtedly heard of the "fight-or-flight" response, which is sometimes called the stress response. The fight-or-flight response is our body's prehistoric method of dealing with stress. It is the mechanism that enabled our ancestors to escape from a saber-toothed tiger, kill a woolly mammoth or today allows a grandmother, in the throes of a terrible accident, to lift a car off her grandchild. Without it, we would not be here today. The stress response is regulated by the sympathetic nervous system and it kicks in automatically without your even thinking about it.

When you are exposed to a stressful situation, the adrenal glands, located on top of the kidneys, begin to pump out stress hormones to help our bodies cope with immediate danger, and prepare for extreme exertion. Our blood pressure rises, our hearts beat faster, our blood is made to clot more easily in the event we are injured, and the flow of blood is routed from the digestive system to the muscles where it is needed to fuel our escape or help us hunt. As all of this is happening, stress hormones called epinephrine (adrenaline) and corticosteroids send blood sugar levels soaring to provide turbo charging fuel that can be burned anaerobically, that is, without oxygen. This is fortunate since under stress and heavy exertion we may not be able to breathe fast enough to supply sufficient oxygen to burn fat. You burn sugar very quickly as you run for your life to get away from a chasing tiger. When the immediate danger and stress are over, you cells should revert back to fat burning, and your body should get back to normal.

What happens when your body continually uses sugar as its primary fuel? The resulting leptin resistance will lock you in sugar burning mode, simulating the "stressed out," fight-or-flight mode. Even though you may not know it, your diet becomes one of the biggest "stressors" in your life, constantly triggering your sympathetic nervous system, whether or not there is an actual danger or stress. You are constantly in the "fight-or-flight," turbo-charged mode and will undergo more and more wear and tear. You will, as would your car engine if continually revved, quickly wear out, age, become diseased, and die.

The vicious cycle born from leptin resistance can have a catastrophic effect on every organ system in the body, seriously compromising health. Fat begins to accumulate in places where this should not happen, such as around the waist or midline. This common condition, known as midline adiposity or commonly as "the apple shape," is a major cause of insulin resistance. The fat that you can see on your body is only the tip of the iceberg. The fat that you don't see can be even more dangerous. Fat deposits accumulate around and within internal organs

WHY YOU WANT TO BE
A FAT BURNER, NOT A SUGAR BURNER

Some of you may be thinking, I may eat a lot of starchy carbohydrates, but at the same meal, I am also eating protein and fat. Why am I just burning sugar and storing fat? It's a good question, and it gets to the heart of the vicious cycle.

Let's assume that you are following the current dietary recommendations that tell you to eat more than half of your daily calories in the form of carbohydrate. You fill your plate with a cup or so of pasta (carbs), topped with meatballs (primarily protein and fat), and some tomato sauce and cheese (more protein and fat). From the moment the pasta enters your mouth, it begins to be broken down into simple sugar. Your body can only store a small amount of sugar at a time in the form of glycogen, which is stored in muscle and liver. What happens to the rest? What's not stored as glycogen is burned off as quickly as possible, forcing you to burn sugar, but your cells can only burn so much off at a time. What happens to the rest of the sugar that isn't being stored or burned? It is converted into saturated fat, and we know where that goes (in all the places that you don't want it: your hips, thighs, abdomen, and dangling from your upper arms).

Your cells are busily burning off sugar for fuel, but what about the protein and fat in your meal? Some of the protein is taken up by your cells for repair and maintenance, but your cells can only utilize a small amount of protein at a time. Excess protein is turned into sugar and stored as saturated fat. (That's *more* fat in your tummy, hips, abdomen, upper arms, etc.) Your cells don't need to burn it for fuel—they're still burning off all the sugar from your plateful of pasta.

That leaves just the fat (from the meat and the cheese). Remember, your cells are hardwired to burn sugar first, so if your cells are burning off lots of sugar, the fat in your meal is going to be stored away as. . . . MORE FAT.

Furthermore, your cells get accustomed to burning a particular fuel. When you are younger, your metabolism is more flexible, and you can switch fuels more easily. As you get older, if your cells are used to burning sugar, they will continue to burn sugar, not fat, when they need fuel. You will need to burn almost every gram of sugar that you've eaten before you can burn off significant amounts of fat.

such as the liver, which cause the liver to become even more insulin resistant. This triggers the liver to produce even more glucose, raising blood sugar, and causing a further rise in insulin and leptin, and further insulin resistance and leptin resistance. Some of that extra fat also accumulates inside the arteries, which increases your risk of heart attack. It is the start of yet another vicious cycle culminating in diabetes, obesity, heart disease, and early death.

Being a constant sugar burner is not a good thing. Even when you're asleep, your body will continue to burn sugar. Once your cells deplete the sugar stored in your liver, they will break down protein from your muscle and even bone to burn as sugar. As long as there is sugar to be had, and your hormones are telling you not to burn fat, your cells won't dig into your fat stores no matter how many pounds of excess fat you have waiting to be burned. As long as you continue to eat a high carbohydrate, high sugar, or excess protein diet, your body will continue burning sugar and storing fat. You will require your sugar fix, and you will remain leptin resistant and stay hungry as a result of your brain's inability to "hear" leptin.

In order to break this vicious cycle, you need to retrain the brain to instruct the cells to burn fat as the body's primary fuel. That is what the Rosedale Diet is all about. It teaches your cells to burn off excess fat from your tummy, your thighs, your rear end, and from other places where you don't want it, such as your arteries. As a bonus, you won't get hungry because your cells are being well fed and properly nourished. You will feel better, you will look better, and you will be healthier.

■ IN HIS OWN WORDS ■

J. P., AGE 65
"I'm a younger man now than I was ten years ago."

I was sick, overweight, and depressed, and had been for years. I was aging rapidly. I would say to myself, "This week I feel much older than I felt last week." I felt as if I was dying, and I had only just turned sixty! I was a top executive for a huge multinational and I was under a great deal of stress. I felt that I had to retire. I was a nervous eater, and just kept eating and eating. I had gained a ton of weight in a relatively short time. I was eating all the wrong food. I'd eat a bagel for breakfast, I'd snack on crackers and peanut butter all day, and I'd always order dessert when I went out to eat. I wasn't paying attention to what I was eating. I had high blood pressure. I was taking antidepressants and was suffering terribly from allergies, so I took allergy medicine every day.

Within the first month of starting on Ron's diet, I lost ten pounds and was off my antidepressants. I didn't need these drugs anymore; I felt great. Within a year, I lost fifty pounds and my blood pressure is now normal. My insulin level dropped from 69 to 10, which is great. My energy level is off the charts. I no longer need my allergy medication—I had been taking it for forty-five years. I mean, that's phenomenal. I've never been hungry on this diet. I've always had lots to eat and it's easy to follow. Ron talks a lot about de-aging your body. All I can tell you is that this strategy seems to be working for me—I'm a younger man now than I was ten years ago.

chapter four

How the Rosedale Diet Can Keep You Young

Once you begin following the Rosedale Diet, you will see how quickly the fat will melt off your body, leaving you well toned, sleek, and strong. What is less obvious is the amazing effect of the Rosedale Diet on your body chemistry, and how it literally "de-ages" your body, giving you the very real possibility of a longer, healthier life span.

Since ancient times, we humans have been searching for the fountain of youth, the secret to living a longer life, free of frailty and the diseases of aging. Ironically, the key to longevity has been right under our noses, only until very recently, we did not have the tools to see it. The good news is, we now have the genetic footprint showing us the way to extend our life span, and enjoy those extra decades in health and vitality. We now know the common denominators that are apparently found in all living beings—worms, mice, monkeys, or even humans— that can allow them to defy the odds and live beyond their expected life span. The even better news is, you don't have to be born with the right genes to live a longer, healthier life. By following the Rosedale Diet, you can actually make your body decades younger, and turn back the clock to a time when you weren't weighed down by all that extra fat, or when you didn't suffer from diabetes or heart disease. My patients have done it, and so can you.

Much of what we know about longevity is derived from studies of humans and animals who have broken the age barrier for their species. Every species has a different potential life span. The longest-lived flies may survive only a few days, mice a couple of years, and dogs for one or two decades, depending on their size. Humans currently have the potential to live 120 years, but virtually no one actually does. The average life expectancy today is around eighty, which is impressive, but nowhere near our full potential.

Growing in ranks, yet still few in number, are the exceptional group of people who live to be 100 or more years old. Scattered throughout the world, these centenarians are providing scientists with a living laboratory from which they can unravel the secrets of longevity.

It would be easy to dismiss longevity merely as a function of the genetic lottery, but we know that this isn't necessarily true. A second and equally rich source of information on longevity has come from the studies of laboratory animals put on calorie-restricted diets. Since the 1930s, dozens of species—microscopic worms, assorted rodents, and more recently, rhesus monkeys, fellow primates that are closely related to humans—have been fed calorie-restricted diets. These animals are fed about one-third fewer calories than normal, but they're not starved; they're given a nutrient enriched diet. These animals virtually always live longer—30 to 80 percent longer. This would be the equivalent of a human living to be 160 to 220 years old!

Not only do they live longer, but they are also healthier, more energetic and look years younger than noncalorie-restricted animals. These longer-lived animals have nearly identical genes as their peers who died younger. The only discernible difference is their diet. How could anybody with this knowledge deny the extraordinary power of diet on health?

At first glance, human centenarians would appear to have very little in common with calorie-restricted animals. There is no evidence that centenarians followed a particular diet, or even had particularly healthy lifestyles. Some centenarians smoked (the oldest known person—one woman who lived to be 122 years old—had smoked for most of her life!), some did not, some exercised regularly, some did not, some were careful eaters, and some ate whatever they wished.

Calorie-restricted animals share a particular metabolic profile—I call it the Longevity Profile—that distinguishes them from their peers who die younger and sicker. In nearly every study, the longest-lived animals share the following traits:

- Low fasting leptin levels
- Low fasting insulin levels
- Reduction in fasting glucose
- Lower body temperature
- Low percentage of body fat
- Reduced thyroid levels
- Low triglycerides (a type of fat in blood)

My patients, even the sickest ones, achieve the Longevity Profile within weeks of following the Rosedale Diet (and believe me, they're not starving! Just look at the menus starting on page 118 if you don't believe me). Calorie-restricted animals may not have been born with the Longevity Profile, but their diet enabled them to re-create it. In other words, eating less has reprogrammed their genes to extend their lives. Centenarians come by the Longevity Profile naturally. It may be encoded in their genes, because regardless of lifestyle, they live longer. They may have been born lucky, but you don't have to be. As far as health and longevity is concerned, you can make your own luck.

■ GENES VERSUS DIET

Some of you may be confused by the notion that genes can be altered through diet or by any other means. After all, didn't we learn in biology class that genes are passed from one generation to the other, and that we don't have any say about which genes we inherit, or what they do in our bodies? As it turns out, this is only partly true. We do inherit all our 22,000 genes (as of last count) from our parents, but that doesn't mean that our destiny is predetermined before birth. All 22,000 genes are not operating at the same time—most remain dormant. Only a fraction of our genes are ever activated, meaning that the rest of our genes have no apparent effect on us. Genes can be "turned on" or "turned off" depending on a wide variety of factors. In science, we talk about genes "expressing" themselves, which simply means making themselves heard in your body. Genes tell your cells how to behave. For example, you may have inherited a gene that makes you prone to develop a certain type of diabetes, but unless you are exposed to a particular environmental toxin (for example, excess sugar in your diet), that gene may never be activated or given an opportunity to "express" itself. The good things that you do for yourself can also have a positive effect on whether or not a "bad" gene can cause mischief. For example, you may be carrying a gene for cancer, or heart disease, or even for depression, but if you eat the right diet, you have a good shot at avoiding these problems. For years, I have told my patients with a family history of diabetes that I don't care if every relative they have going back many generations has had diabetes—they will not become diabetic if they follow my program, and you can't find too many promises (or for that matter, any) in medicine.

From the studies of calorie-restricted animals, it is clear that diet, specifically, eating fewer calories, can have a profound impact on genetic expression. The question is, why would eating less add so many more years to your life? Many of you have heard of the Human Genome Project, the heroic effort started in 1990 to map and identify every single human gene. From the Human Genome Project, we learned a surprising fact: Our genes are very similar to those of almost every other species on earth. If you compared human genes with the genes of primitive organisms such as worms, you would find that we share about 70 percent of their genes. If you compared human genes with chimpanzees, you would find that our genes would be almost identical, or more precisely, about 99.44 percent the same. Yet there is a vast difference between humans and worms and even between humans and monkeys, despite our close genetics. Clearly, genes are expressed differently from species to species, which is what distinguishes our species from others.

Despite the obvious differences between species, we share a common history that is literally written in our genes. Each of us carries a huge genetic library that dates back to our earliest, primordial past. As our species evolved through the ages, we may add new genes to that library, but we do not eliminate the old genes. Like dated volumes in a library gathering dust, we may store the old genes away, but we hold on to them in case we ever need to use them again.

■ LONGEVITY ISN'T "NATURAL"

Within the billions of years that life has evolved on earth, we may have become smarter, more complicated creatures than our single-celled predecessors, but the fact is, we are here for pretty much the same reason. As Mother Nature sees it, whether you are a single-celled organism, a multicelled nematode, a bird, a dog, a cat, or a human, you are here for the primary purpose to reproduce and pass your precious genes (the library of life) on to the next generation. After that, you're expendable. My patients are shocked when I tell them that there is nothing "natural" about trying to live as long a life as possible. You may want to hang around to be a healthy 120 and spend your last decades playing with your great-grandchildren, writing your novel, or traveling the world, but Mother Nature has other ideas. Mother Nature's primary concern is to keep you alive long enough to reproduce, and maybe a bit longer after that to care for your young. That's it. Some scientists believe that our cavemen ancestors followed an ideal diet for our health and longevity because they ate the "pure" and "natural" diet that we all evolved from. In reality, the so-called "paleolithic diet" followed by cavemen was not necessarily ideal for long-term health; in fact, it was sort of random. Cavemen ate whatever Mother Nature made available to them at the time. Keep in mind, Mother Nature didn't give a whit about eating for a long healthy life; she just wanted cavemen to make more baby cavemen. You see why I say there's nothing "natural" about the quest for longevity? If anything, in order to achieve longevity, you have to circumvent Mother Nature and consider some "unnatural" alternatives. By that I mean you have to "trick" Mother Nature at her own game.

Nature has very ingenious ways to help a species survive. When food is scarce, as it often was for our more primitive ancestors, in order to ensure the survival of a species, nature developed a method of keeping an organism alive through times of famine so that it could reproduce at a later, more opportune time. Reduced food intake turns on genes that protect the body against aging, allowing it to hopefully outlive the famine. Instead of spending lots of scarce energy to make babies that couldn't survive, the body focuses its energy on maintaining and repairing itself. As soon as there is enough food available to support effective reproduction, the body switches gears and reduces its emphasis on maintenance and repair and directs its energy toward reproduction.

When you are in maintenance and repair mode, the body's "body shop" is revved up and ready to go. Calorie-restricted animals have measurably higher levels of key chemicals that allow for extended life, protect cells from damage, and promote repair.

▪ LEPTIN IS THE KEY

You don't have to starve yourself to turn on the maintenance and repair switch. Following the Rosedale Diet will do the same good things for your body. How does it work? Leptin is a key player (perhaps in concert with insulin) in the evolutionary tug of war between whether the body should concentrate on reproduction or maintenance and repair. In mammals, high leptin levels are the evolutionary signal that you have enough stored food around to successfully reproduce. Therefore, there's no reason for your genes to turn on the maintenance and repair mechanisms to keep you around much longer. In contrast, I suspect keeping your leptin levels low "tricks" Mother Nature into thinking that food is scarce, even when it may not be. Your body's "body shop" works overtime to keep you around so that you can reproduce far into the future. (Of course, this doesn't prevent a woman from becoming menopausal, but it can still keep her body in more youthful condition.) Lowering leptin levels is a sign to turn on our ancient instructions for maintenance and repair to keep you healthy. In calorie-restricted animals, eating less turns on the repair and maintenance genes in their bodies, giving them a longer life. For reasons we don't quite understand, centenarians are blessed with genes that also turn on these same maintenance and repair mechanisms, enabling them to live longer. You can enjoy the same advantage by following the Rosedale Diet.

As a "master hormone," leptin controls all the other biomarkers of the Longevity Profile. If your leptin levels rise to unhealthy levels, making you leptin resistant, you will not have the optimal Longevity Profile. Your insulin levels will be higher, your body will run at too high a temperature, your blood glucose level will be higher than it should be, and you will have excess body fat. The bottom line: Your body will not switch into "maintenance and repair mode" and your cells will not be maintained in optimal condition. Instead of adding years to your life, you could be taking them away.

Each of the biomarkers in the Longevity Profile works synergistically to create a favorable environment in your body that turns up maintenance and repair. Each biomarker also has independent benefits, which I describe below.

■ THE BENEFITS OF LOW INSULIN

If there is a known single marker for a longer life span, as they are finding in the centenarian and laboratory animal studies, it is insulin sensitivity, or low insulin levels. When your cells are not sensitive to insulin, your insulin levels go up. What is the purpose of insulin? If you ask your doctor, he or she will tell you that it's to lower blood sugar, but I believe that's just a trivial side effect. Insulin's evolutionary purpose is to store excess energy for future times of need. It lowers blood glucose levels for the purpose of storing it away, not regulating it. For our ancestors, this was a good thing. Remember, our ancestors survived on whatever food they could find, and they did not typically find food that elevated glucose. They ate some fruit when it was in season, but much of the sugar was burned in gathering it. High glucose was not a big problem back then! Very often, they were forced to survive for days, weeks or even months on little food. Insulin helped our ancestors store away nutrients for the proverbial rainy day when they would need it.

• • •

Our diet is completely different today. Food is plentiful, and high glucose is the norm, not the exception. As a result, our insulin levels are typically much higher than they were among our ancestors. When your cells are constantly bombarded with insulin, they become insulin resistant, meaning they stop hearing insulin's important message. Moreover, excess insulin can damage your cells. In fact, insulin resistance may be a defense mechanism on the part of cells to protect against the toxic effects of excess insulin. This creates a hormonal derangement that has a catastrophic effect on your metabolism.

Makes You Fat. One of the first and potentially deadliest effects of becoming insulin resistant is excess weight gain, which leads to obesity, as discussed in Chapter 3. There is a particular deadly pattern to weight gain caused by insulin resistance: First you get obese, then you become diabetic. Why? Not all cells become insulin resistant at the same time. Liver cells may be the first to become insulin resistant. Since one of insulin's effects is to suppress production of sugar by the liver, if the liver is no longer listening to insulin, it is going to make a lot of sugar. Eventually muscle cells will become insulin resistant, too. Then they can't burn the sugar that was manufactured by the liver, and as we know, if sugar isn't burned off, it is stored as fat. Your fat cells are among the last to become insulin resistant, which is a real problem because insulin promotes the making and storage of fat. Thanks to insulin, all that excess sugar that hasn't been burned off is now socked away as fat! Eventually, your fat cells will become insulin resistant, and you can then stop making all that fat, but then you have no place to put the excess sugar and it starts building up in your blood, and you finally become diabetic. Until your fat cells become insulin resistant, you get fatter and fatter, and that is the fat that you see on your body. The end result is severe obesity. Some people plateau at 200 pounds, some at 300 pounds, and a rare few go beyond that.

Bad for Your Heart. Excess insulin and insulin resistance do a great deal of damage throughout your body. Insulin stores magnesium in cells, which is important because magnesium inside the cell helps relax muscles. Insulin signaling results in the inability to properly store magnesium. When you lose magnesium, your blood vessels constrict, making it harder for your blood to flow throughout your body. As a result, your blood pressure rises and your coronary arteries could spasm, resulting in a heart attack. Also, without magnesium and proper insulin signaling, you can't properly manufacture important fatty acids such as EPA and DHA, which are vital to your health.

Excess insulin also causes retention of sodium, which causes fluid retention, elevates blood pressure, and can lead to congestive heart failure. Studies have shown that if you drip insulin into an artery of a dog, the artery will become blocked with plaque after several months. Plaque buildup in arteries can deprive the heart of blood and oxygen and eventually lead to a heart attack.

Did you know that heart attacks are much more likely to happen after a high carbohydrate meal than after a high fat meal? The immediate effects of raising your blood sugar from a high carb meal is to raise insulin and leptin. That in turn triggers the "stress response" which will cause arterial spasm, constriction of the arteries and arrhythmia or irregular heartbeat.

Cancer Link. In most species of calorie-restricted animals, life span increases primarily as a result of a reduction in cancer rates (cancer being the number one killer in most animals). This is not surprising. Insulin is closely related to another hormone, IGF-1, or insulin-like growth factor. As its name implies, IGF's primary function is to promote growth . . . and reproduction. There is a strong link between IGF levels and cancer (which is not much more than excessive cellular reproduction). Because of its molecular similarity to IGF, insulin can trigger the same genetic message, promoting growth and reproduction . . . and cancer. Moreover, there is a highly significant correlation between a diet high in starchy and sugary carbohydrates; elevated insulin levels; and breast, colon, prostate, and pancreatic cancer incidence.

Bad for Your Bones. Elevated insulin is even a risk factor for osteoporosis, the bone-breaking disease characterized by the thinning of bone. Insulin promotes the excretion of calcium in the urine, and calcium is an important mineral component of bone. Simply taking a calcium supplement, as so many doctors advise, isn't going to maintain bone health. If it is in a high insulin environment, the calcium will simply be washed out of the body. (See page 192 for more information on osteoporosis.)

■ LOW FASTING GLUCOSE LEVELS

Why do the longest living humans and animals have low blood sugar levels for their age? First, high blood levels of sugar send leptin levels soaring, as explained earlier. Second, elevated glucose levels are often a reflection of a diet high in nonfiber carbohydrate, which is the equivalent of eating huge amounts of sugar every day. Finally, as noted in earlier chapters, elevated glucose levels can also be a result of eating too much protein, and this is what is so worrisome about the "eat all the protein you want" diets. Eat too much food that raises sugar and insulin levels (including too much protein) and that sugar will be stored as fat around your waist and midline, which puts a strain on the heart.

Ages You. When glucose encounters protein in your body, bad things can happen. In a process called glycation, glucose reacts with protein, resulting in "sticky proteins." This can create sugar-damaged proteins called advanced glycation end products, or AGES for short. When protein is damaged, it cannot function properly or communicate properly with other cells. AGES also promotes excessive inflammation throughout the body. The acronym AGES is quite appropriate, since a high number of these damaged proteins can lead to premature aging. The process of glycation occurs in everyone, but it occurs at a higher rate in people with elevated blood sugar, such as those who are diabetic. Glycation is one of the major reasons why diabetics appear to look so much older than nondiabetics, and suffer the so-called diseases of aging at younger ages than they should.

AGES can cause brown spots or age spots to appear on skin, as well as premature wrinkles. AGES also can wreak havoc on the organs of the body. If the protein in the collagen of the arteries becomes damaged, it can promote the formation of plaque, thereby causing a heart attack. If the collagen in connective tissue becomes riddled with AGES, it could cause arthritis. If the protein in the lens of the eye becomes damaged, it could promote the formation of cataracts and eventual blindness. Glycation can also promote the formation of free radicals, which in excess, can destroy more healthy cells and age the body even faster.

The glycation process has also been linked to the destruction of nerve cells. In the brain, that could eventually lead to Alzheimer's disease and other neurological diseases. Diabetics are at particular risk of peripheral neuropathy, characterized by injury to nerve cells in the toes, feet, legs, and arms. Unfortunately, peripheral neuropathy can be very serious, and can even result in amputation of the affected limb.

Here's yet another reason to lay off starchy food: Heating starches, especially frying them (like French fries and chips) can produce a type of glycated protein called acrilamides, which are potent carcinogens. Acrilamides are so widespread in the food supply that the World Health Organization recently called a special session to discuss this new threat to world health. Limiting starches of any kind, but especially baked and fried starches, is the only way to protect yourself against these cancer-causing agents.

Memory Problems. A recent study showed that people with elevated levels of blood sugar have more memory problems than people with normal blood sugar, regardless of their age. Undoubtedly, this is at least in part due to excess glycation.

Suppresses Immune System. High blood sugar can suppress your immune system, making you more vulnerable to infection. Glucose is very similar in molecular structure to vitamin C, so similar, in fact, that your cells could easily mistake one for the other. Immune cells require higher amounts of vitamin C to gobble up invading bacteria, viruses, and cancer cells. If there is a lot of glucose floating around, your immune cells could take in glucose instead of vitamin C, which will impair their function.

▪ LOWER BODY TEMPERATURE

Why would having a lower body temperature extend your life? Body temperature is a reflection of your metabolic rate. Metabolism is the way your body transforms energy into the work of life. Thyroid hormone helps control metabolic rate, and leptin controls the thyroid. How many times have you seen commercials for weight loss products that promise to "turn up" your metabolism? In reality, these terms are very misleading. I tell my patients that they should be much more concerned about the *quality* of their metabolism than the *quantity*. What you really want is a more efficient metabolism that runs your body without causing a lot of wear and tear.

Heat Is Wasted Energy. Thermogenic literally means "creating heat," and contrary to what manufacturers of so-called "thermogenic aids" say in their commercials, running "hotter" is not good, and is actually very bad for you. Heat can have a decidedly negative effect on your cells. We do require some heat; obviously, we don't want to freeze, but excess heat is very harmful and accelerates aging. Your body is forced to work harder to get rid of the potentially disruptive heat (you sweat, your heart pumps faster and the arterioles in your skin dilate) and you are wasting energy that could otherwise be going toward maintenance and repair. Think in terms of your car. For example, let's say that your car stalls and sputters at every stoplight. You take your car to your mechanic, and he says, "No problem, I'll just turn up the idle," which is the equivalent of saying, "No problem, I'll just turn up your thyroid production." Your car no longer stalls at the stoplight, but you're idling at 2,000 rpm. How long is your engine going to last? It's going to overheat and need more repairs, and you're going to get poor mileage. It will be headed shortly for the salvage yard. A better approach is to use clean spark plugs, make sure that fuel lines are clean, and that the timing is good—in other words, make sure the car can efficiently and correctly turn the energy from gasoline into proper function. Then your car will work better. You'll get much better mileage, better pickup, and you won't put as much stress on the engine. To a car, better mileage is really equal to longevity. By running cooler, cleaner, and more efficiently, you've made your car healthier and extended its life.

The same rules apply to all life—including your life. Flowers are kept cool at the florist for good reason. Keep them in a warm environment and they wilt faster. Simply turning up metabolism is not going to extend your life, or even make you a better fat burner (unless you have thyroid disease and *abnormally* low thyroid function). Increasing heat is wasting energy. Instead of wasting all that energy as heat, you could be directing more of it to maintenance and repair, that is, keeping you in a more youthful state. If you have a poor metabolism, if you are stuck in sugar burning mode, increasing metabolism will just accelerate the rate at which you are burning sugar and tearing down your muscle and bone. People who are hyperthyroid—who have excess production of thyroid hormone—often have osteoporosis. Thyroid hormone may control the rate of metabolism, but not the *quality* of metabolism. There is a big difference. Leptin, in turn, helps to control the thyroid and along with insulin controls the quality of metabolism.

I am delighted when I see a patient's thyroid hormone level go down, as it typically does on my program, as their energy, their "pickup," increases. It means that their body is functioning efficiently, more energy is directed toward keeping them healthy and alive, and precious "energy" is not being wasted in the form of excess heat. (Reducing your level of thyroid hormone in this healthy way is not the same thing as having a low thyroid level due to a diseased thyroid—or hypothyroidism. In the case of hypothyroidism, your thyroid gland is stuck in low gear and is functioning poorly. In contrast, on the Rosedale Diet, your thyroid gland works very well and it doesn't have to work as hard.) You can slow down metabolism, yet still be more "energized" if you turn it into high quality metabolism. That is what the Rosedale Diet does.

■ LOW TRIGLYCERIDES

Low triglycerides are generally a marker that you are metabolizing fat efficiently, and in all likelihood you will have an easier time burning fat as your primary fuel, and that insulin and leptin are working well in your body.

■ OBESITY SHORTENS YOUR LIFE

Sure, having low body fat will make you look a lot better in a bathing suit, but there are even more compelling reasons why you want to stay lean. The more fat you burn, the healthier you are going to be, and the longer you are going to live. Lean bodies live longer. Carrying around a lot of excess fat is detrimental to your long-term survival. The human body did not evolve to run well weighed down by fat! How could a body loaded with excess fat have the speed or agility to escape a predator or run after prey? From a purely evolutionary standpoint, too much fat is bad.

Numerous studies have confirmed that obesity can shorten your life and make you more vulnerable to the diseases of aging at younger and younger ages. Unfortunately, the obesity epidemic especially among children and teenagers is showing the devastating consequences of poor diet. For the first time in history, doctors are routinely diagnosing type 2 diabetes in obese children, a condition that is called adult-onset diabetes because it is not supposed to occur in children. They may be children, but their bodies are stuck in accelerated aging mode, which does not bode well for their long-term health or survival.

If You're Fat, You're Burning Sugar. At any age, if you have a high percentage of body fat, it is a sign that you are not burning fat, but storing it. If you are not burning fat, you are burning sugar, and that means that you are burning through your muscle, and protein in your bones (since you can make sugar out of them). You are not only aging your body faster, but you are dooming yourself to grow old in a weak, frail body.

Leptin-Insulin Resistance. Remember, the vicious cycle I discussed in Chapter 3? The more fat cells you make, the more leptin you will produce, and the more leptin resistant you become. Your body loses its ability to control hunger, you overeat, and make more fat and fat cells. On a more profound level, high levels of leptin signal to your brain that there is plenty of nourishment around for reproduction, and no need to live long and prosper. Genes that up-regulate maintenance and repair get turned down.

Body Fat Promotes Diabetes. Fat has a way of congregating in places where you don't want it. For example, if you are leptin resistant, excess fat is often stored around your waist, right by your liver. Excess fat in and around your liver disrupts insulin signaling, leading to insulin resistance, diabetes, and a downward spiral that ages you before your time. Fat can also clog your arteries, which can cause a heart attack.

Body Fats, Hormones, and Cancer. Since dozens of hormones are made and stored in fat, excess fat can disturb the normal hormonal balance in the body, which may increase the risk of hormone sensitive cancers. Higher levels of estrogen due to more body fat explains why obese women are at greater risk of breast cancer than normal weight women. In men, too much body fat increases the activity of an enzyme called aromatase which converts testosterone into estrogen. This leads to lower testosterone levels, higher estrogen levels, and an increased risk of prostate enlargement, prostate cancer, and obesity. Not to mention the fact that it makes men flabby!

▪ IN HIS OWN WORDS ▪

S. L., AGE 54

"I don't need to eat food for comfort anymore, I take comfort in how I look and how I feel."

I went to see Ron because I had diabetes and high blood pressure, and was taking a drug called Glucotrol (which increases insulin production by the islet cells in the pancreas) and medicine to lower my blood pressure. I didn't like being on all this medicine, and I was also very overweight. I weighed close to 300 pounds; I'm now down to 220. When I started on the program, the first thing Ron did was take me off the Glucotrol. He said, "You know, you don't need to make more insulin, you need to make better use of the insulin that you already have." He was right. When he tested my insulin level, it was elevated.

I've been a police officer for more than thirty years, and I'm going to retire soon. Cops get into some real bad eating habits. You stop and grab a doughnut and you don't think about eating healthy stuff. You eat for comfort. You eat to relieve the stress of the job.

On Ron's program, I lost weight fairly quickly, and my blood pressure was down to normal without drugs. I've been able to maintain my weight loss and I never feel deprived. Whereas before when I went on a diet, I would think, "Oh gosh, I need a slice of pizza," I don't think that way anymore. Eating for my health as well as my appearance and weight has just made all the difference in the world in how I look and feel.

Ron has also got me to do some weight lifting—not too much. I do a lot of reps with a light weight. He explained to me how weight training makes the cells more sensitive to insulin, and it's just amazing what it did for me. I don't need to eat food for comfort anymore; I take comfort in looking great and being healthy. There's nothing better than being able to buy clothes right off the rack in normal sizes. I'm down to a 38 pant. I don't have to shop in the big and tall man store anymore. It's just fantastic. I kept a couple of my old, baggy pants as reminders of what I used to look like and it's all the incentive I need to stay on the program.

part · two

Making the Rosedale Diet Work for You

chapter ▪ five

Why Good Fat
Does a Body Good

W hat makes food taste great? What makes you feel full and satisfied? What is the food you need to eat in order to burn fat?
Surprise! The answer, in a word, is FAT . . . and yes, it's great
for your body as long as it's the right kind of fat.

For decades, we've been told that fat—any kind of fat—is
bad stuff that clogs up your arteries, destroys your heart and
adds extra pounds to your body. It's been drummed into our
heads that fat makes us fat. We listened to the experts and
stopped eating high fat foods like nuts, fatty fish, avocados,
and healthy oils and loaded up on low fat, high carbohydrate
foods like pasta and cereal. Ironically, while we were eliminating natural fat from our diet, we were filling up with man-
made fats like margarine and processed cooking oils, which
were touted by the food industry as heart healthy. And what
happened? We are in the midst of the worst epidemic of obesity in recorded history, type 2 diabetes is now the most preva-
lent disease of our time, and heart disease is on the rise.

The experts were flat-out wrong. ALL FAT IS NOT BAD
AND ALL FAT IS NOT THE SAME. When it comes to fat,
it's not so simple.

- Some types of fat are bad for you all of the time, and some types of fat are bad for you only some of the time. The health effects of fat often depend on what you eat with it.
- Good fats are essential for maintaining proper weight and optimal health.
- If you cut out fat and replace it with starchy or sweet carbohydrates, you will end up burning sugar and making and storing fat. That is what will make you fat.
- Margarine and most vegetable oils (especially the ones used in cooking and processed foods) are worse for you than butter.

As it turns out, fat is an essential nutrient. We need fat. Wild animals covet fat. Sharks are much more likely to eat fat animals such as seals as opposed to lean animals. (Yet another reason to become lean!) Mice go for the cheese. They feel better and they are healthier when they eat fat, and they can go for longer periods of time without eating. I saw the lure of fat firsthand when I was eating lunch with my family at an outdoor café in San Diego a number of years ago. Seagulls kept trying to attack a basket of bread that had been placed on our table. The waiter kept "shooing them" off with a broom. My sister and mother laughed and said to the waiter that they were just trying to get the bread. The waiter said, "Oh no, they are trying to get the butter—they always go for the butter." I was struck by how all animals (including humans) need and crave fat, and how ridiculous it is to try to cut fat out of the human diet.

I'm not giving you carte blanche to eat any kind of fat. As I teach my patients, it is critical to know the difference between good fat and bad fat, and how to get the right kind of fat in your diet. When it comes to eating fat, the *quality* of fat you eat is far more important than obsessing over the *quantity*. To me, most of nutrition boils down to what kinds of fat to eat. Fat can be your best friend . . . or your worst enemy.

■ THE THREE KINDS OF FAT

There are in general three different types of fat: saturated fat, poly-unsaturated fat, and monounsaturated fat. All fat is made up of chains of fatty acids, but the different types of fatty acids have different mo-lecular configurations, and act very differently in the body.

Polyunsaturated Fat. Remember all those margarine commercials on television claiming that the polyunsaturated fat in margarine could pro-tect you against heart disease? Turns out, it was only half true. We now know that not all polyunsaturated fat is the same: Some are good, some are harmless, and some—like the fat used in most brands of margarine—can be downright dangerous. In some cases, polyunsatu-rated fat can be much more harmful than, for instance, the saturated fat found in butter.

Polyunsaturated fat is found primarily in vegetable oils such as omega-6 fatty acids, (soy, sesame, sunflower, safflower, corn, cotton-seed, peanut) seeds, and margarine. The essential fatty acids—omega-3 (found in fatty fish) and omega-6—are polyunsaturated fat. Though some omega-6 fat is essential to your health, excess omega-6 fat can also be very hazardous to your health. Two other polyunsaturated fats—trans fatty acids and hydrogenated fats—commonly found in processed foods, can also be hazardous to your health and I want you to avoid them (entirely if possible). When it comes to polyunsaturated fat, you must make the right choices or suffer the consequences.

The downside of all polyunsaturated fats is that they are unstable, that is, they are easily oxidized, which can promote the formation of po-tentially toxic chemicals called free radicals. In limited amounts free radicals are fine; in fact, they are necessary for our survival. In excess, however, free radicals can destroy healthy cells and promote disease and premature aging. If you eat a diet high in polyunsaturated fat, you may end up loading your body with free radicals. Heating polyunsatu-rated oil accelerates the formation of free radicals (in frying pans and in your body). Take note: Most fast-food restaurants and Asian restaurants fry food in polyunsaturated oil, usually soy oil because it is so cheap.

Every time you eat fried food, you are eating a hefty serving of free radicals. (You are not defenseless against free radicals. You can control the potentially damaging effect of free radicals by taking an ample amount of fat soluble antioxidant supplements, and by eating a diet filled with vegetables, which contain natural antioxidants. For more information on supplements, see page 134.)

Saturated Fat. This fat is primarily found in grain-fed animals, including meat, lamb, and dairy products from grain-fed animals (milk, cheese, lard, and butter) and to a lesser extent, poultry and fish. Although derived from plants, coconut oil is also high in saturated fat, but of a different kind, that may even have health benefits.

Why are grain-fed animals so high in saturated fat? Animals, like us, turn the grain that they eat into sugar, and then into saturated fat. The fat in grain-fed animals is really second generation carbohydrates. It has been known for hundreds of years that feeding grain to animals makes them fat. That is why cattle go to feed lots before they are sold—to make them fat as fast as possible. That is also what grain feeding does to us!

Unlike polyunsaturated fat, saturated fat tends to be hard at room temperature. Studies have suggested that a diet high in saturated fat may promote heart disease and insulin resistance. This is true, although some types of polyunsaturated fat can be just as bad—even worse. Saturated fat does have one advantage over polyunsaturated fats, even the good fats: It is not easily oxidized and therefore does not promote free radical production in the body. I still don't advise people to eat a huge amount of saturated fat—not if you want to lose fat. Most of the fat stored in your body is saturated fat, and, in general, it is the toughest fat to burn. If you are looking to shed pounds, it is best to limit (not eliminate) your intake of saturated fat.

Monounsaturated Fat. Monounsaturated fat (omega-9 fatty acids) is not an essential fat, but it's an important fat. It's found primarily in olive oil, avocado, and nuts. The highly touted Mediterranean diet, which appears to reduce the risk of heart disease and some forms of cancer, is rich in olive oil. In Italy and Greece, olive oil is routinely used instead of

FAT RELIEVES STRESS

You think that your life is stressful? Just try living in a cage! Laboratory animals are at high risk of suffering from stress disorders and premature death. A high fat diet has been shown to alleviate the negative, life-shortening effects of stress in laboratory animals. The same appears to be true for humans. Eating a low fat diet can promote depression and anxiety in humans. To me, the cure is obvious: Eat more good fat!

butter, margarine, or processed oils to cook and flavor food. I don't attribute all the health benefits of the Mediterranean diet to olive oil; there are numerous other healthy diet and lifestyle habits of people in that part of the world. For example, in Mediterranean countries, lunch is the big meal of the day, and dinner is a light repast. And though they may eat bread and pasta, their portions are smaller than the typical American portion, and they eat far more seafood and vegetables than Americans eat. Their lifestyle is more relaxing as well. Nevertheless, there is a link between the consumption of olive oil and a decrease in the standard degenerative diseases typical of the Western diet. There is also a link between the consumption of nuts (one of the few foods that contain monounsaturated fats) and a decreased risk of heart disease, a fact that kept popping up in population studies trying to link fat consumption to heart disease, and that confounded researchers convinced that all fat was bad. The experts called contradictory findings "paradoxes," including the well-known "French paradox," and the "Eskimo paradox": Those populations of people ate diets very high in fat, but had a very low incidence of heart disease.

I've reviewed the studies on monounsaturated fat and I'm still not convinced that monounsaturated or omega-9 fat has any special health properties, yet people who eat monounsaturated fats seem to be protected against certain common diseases. Olive oil and nuts do contain beneficial antioxidants that could offer some protection against disease, but I don't think that's the real story. I believe that the major benefit of monounsaturated fat is what it is not. It is not *bad* for you and doesn't have any of the negative effects of other oils. Even "good fats" can promote excess amounts of free radicals if eaten in excess. I believe that monounsaturated fats are mostly benign and have a neutral effect on the body, and therefore, offer essentially a trouble-free fuel.

Sesame, sunflower, corn, and safflower oil contain some monounsaturated oil, but contain mostly omega-6 oil. Therefore, I advise people to stick to olive oil unless they don't like the flavor. If you really can't stand the taste of olive oil, you can use avocado or canola oil.

■ ESSENTIAL FATTY ACIDS

Essential fatty acids are polyunsaturated fats that cannot be produced by the body, and must be obtained through food. Your body cannot function without an adequate amount of essential fatty acids. They provide the raw materials for hormones, and are a major component of cell membranes. As I will explain, these fats can even behave like hormones in the body.

There are two kinds of essential fatty acids: omega-3 fatty acids and omega-6 fatty acids. Omega-3 fatty acids include docosahexaenoic acid (DHA) and eicosapentaenoic acid (EPA). DHA in particular has been linked to a reduced risk of depression and is critical for normal brain function. Several studies have shown that people who eat diets rich in omega-3 fatty acids have a reduced risk of heart disease and stroke. The modern diet tends to be heavy in omega-6 fatty acids (primarily from vegetable oil used in processed foods and cooking), and deficient in omega-3 fatty acids, which are found in cold water fatty fish, deep green vegetables, and to a lesser extent, some nuts. Our hunter-gatherer ancestors had a ratio of omega-6 fatty acids to omega-3 fatty acids of about five to one. Today, that ratio is about twenty-four to one! We are literally bombarding our bodies with omega-6 fatty acids and starving them of omega-3s. Even though omega-6 fatty acids are essential, excess omega-6 fatty acids can promote inflammation, which has been linked to a wide range of diseases including heart disease, cancer, arthritis, and Alzheimer's disease. Diets high in omega-6 fatty acids have been shown to lower the life span of laboratory animals. Moreover, we are compounding the problem by denying our bodies the positive effects of omega-3s, which I outline later.

■ WHY DO WE NEED FAT?

Fat is critical to our survival. Our cell membranes—the protective cover encasing the trillions of cells in the body—are made of fat. The cell membrane is not an inert covering—far from it. The cell membrane is a hotbed of activity. Everything that gets in or out of the cell must pass through the membrane. It is the gatekeeper of the cell. A well-functioning cell membrane is fluid and permeable, that is, it is easy for nutrients to pass into the cell, and waste products to pass out of it.

Whatever fat is in your diet often ends up in your cell membranes. Too much bad fat—saturated fat or trans-fatty acids found in hydrogenated oils—can make a cell membrane rigid and hard, and this will inhibit "flow" of nutrients into the cell. Getting nutrients *into* your cell is the final and most important part of your circulation and is in fact the main purpose of circulation. A nutrient circulating in your bloodstream is in most instances useless, and in some cases harmful, if it cannot get into your cells.

A well-functioning cell membrane is also a "smart" cell membrane. For example, special receptors on the cell membrane "decide" which hormonal signals they will listen to. When you become insulin resistant, for example, insulin receptors on the cell membrane can no longer hear the cues from insulin as well as they should. So the pancreas produces more insulin, which will make you even more insulin resistant, and eventually diabetic. A well-functioning cell membrane is a fundamental key to a healthy and optimally functioning body. In sum, good health depends on high quality cell membranes.

If omega-3 fatty acids are a primary fat in your diet, chances are you will have well-functioning cell membranes. If, on the other hand, you eat a lot of saturated fat or trans-fatty acids, your cell membranes may not function as well.

GOOD FAT CAN'T UNDO THE BAD EFFECTS OF BAD FAT

If you eat a diet very high in saturated fat, taking an omega-3 supplement will not undo all the damage. Saturated fat will crowd out other good fat, so in order to have a cell membrane that contains good fat, you will need to eat a lot more good fat, and a lot less saturated fat.

Omega-6 fatty acids (in commercial oils such as soy and corn oil and most brands of margarine) are often promoted as healthy fat, yet they may be as bad, if not worse, than saturated fat for your cell membranes. These fats are highly vulnerable to free radical attack, which means that when they become incorporated into your cell membranes, they will become free radical magnets. They are also likely to promote inflammation, which can damage healthy cells and spread throughout the body like a fire out of control. Don't eat a lot of them! Although omega-3 fatty acids are also easily oxidized, they have other benefits that far outweigh any disadvantages, as I describe below.

■ THE GOOD NEWS ABOUT OMEGA-3 FATTY ACIDS

Improves Leptin and Insulin Sensitivity

Fish oil can improve insulin sensitivity and leptin sensitivity via its ability to improve membrane flow and function. All the good results I list next are due in large part to the positive effect of fish oil on cell membranes.

TRANS-FATTY ACIDS: UNNATURAL AND UNNECESSARY

Some polyunsaturated fats and margarine undergo a process called hydrogenation to extend their shelf life and make them useful for baking. This process reconfigures the fat molecule, creating a new type of fat called trans-fatty acids. When trans-fatty acids become incorporated into your cell membranes, they make the membranes especially hard and rigid. Trans-fatty acids can disrupt cellular communication, which means that the affected tissues and organs cannot function properly. Trans-fatty acid consumption has been linked to an increased risk of insulin resistance, breast cancer, and heart disease, among other serious health problems.

Your best defense is to avoid trans-fatty acids altogether. This is easier said than done. Trans-fatty acids pop up in the least likely places, from so-called "health food" cereals to packaged baked goods to French fries. *If a food comes in a package, is fried, or contains partially hydrogenated or hydrogenated oils, assume that it contains trans-fatty acids unless the label says otherwise.*

In 2003, the FDA passed a ruling requiring food manufacturers to list the trans-fatty acid content on food labels along with the saturated fat, monounsaturated fat, and polyunsaturated content by 2004. For years, I have been teaching my patients how to calculate the total amount of trans-fatty acids in a particular product. It's not difficult, but it can be a nuisance. To get the total amount of trans-fatty acids, add the total amount of saturated, monounsaturated, and polyunsaturated fat (all listed on the label) and subtract that total from the total fat content listed on the label. Any unaccounted for fat is trans-fatty acids. In the meantime, many food manufacturers are starting to cut back or eliminate trans-fatty acids from their products. As far as I'm concerned, there's no need for trans-fatty acids to be in our food at all. Human life should come before shelf life! Send food manufacturers a message: Don't buy products that contain these dangerous fats.

A WORD ABOUT FLAXSEED OIL

'm frequently asked about flaxseed and flaxseed oil, which in recent years has been touted as a vegetarian source of EPA and DHA, the good fats derived from the omega-3 fatty acids found in fatty fish. In fact, flaxseed does not contain any EPA or DHA. It contains alpha-linolenic acid, which under ideal circumstances can be converted into EPA and DHA in the body. However, many people lack sufficient amounts of the enzymes needed to convert enough linolenic acid into EPA or DHA. The people who need these good fats the most—diabetics, heart patients, and the elderly—may not be able to manufacture much EPA or DHA from flaxseed oil. We evolved eating fish and fish oil, and not flaxseed oil. My advice is, if you are overweight or otherwise at all unhealthy and if you want good fat, you should eat fish and take a fish oil supplement.

Promotes Fat Burning

If you eat the right fat, you will burn fat and lose weight and gain muscle. I've seen this phenomenon in my patients, and it's been proven in the laboratory. Numerous studies have confirmed that when animals are fed a diet rich in omega-3 fatty acids, they gain less weight, stay leaner, and have smaller fat cells than animals fed a diet rich in omega-6 fatty acids (like the diet most Americans eat today). Omega-3 oils seem to turn on the fat-burning metabolic machinery.

Essential for Brain Health

Feed your brain omega-3 fatty acids and you will be smarter, sharper, and happier. More than 70 percent of the dry weight of the human brain is made of fat, and it needs an adequate supply of the right fat to repair and maintain its billions of cells, and to make neurotransmitters, the chemical messengers that help regulate mood, memory, and learning. The best fat for your brain cells is DHA which is found in fatty fish (like salmon and tuna) and supplements. Low blood levels of DHA are associated with brain disorders ranging from depression to Alzheimer's disease to age-related cognitive changes. DHA plays a pivotal role in the production of key brain and nerve cells and is important for good vision. Every activity controlled by the brain—from thinking to learning to running all the organ systems in the body—is dependent on brain cells being able to communicate with one another. DHA provides brain cell membranes with the flexibility necessary for efficient signal transmissions.

DHA is especially important for your mood. In a groundbreaking article published in the *American Journal of Clinical Nutrition,* authors Drs. Joseph R. Hibbeln and Norman Salem Jr., of the National Institutes of Health hypothesize that the increase in depression reported in North America during the twentieth century was probably due to the decrease of DHA in the diet. This hypothesis makes a good deal of sense considering the fact that DHA is vital for the production of neurotransmitters, such as serotonin, which helps regulate mood.

Good for Your Heart

Study after study has shown that fish eaters typically have lower rates of heart disease than non–fish eaters. The heart benefits of omega-3 fatty acids are so well established that even the typically conservative cardiologists are now recommending that some heart patients use fish oil supplements. Omega-3 fatty acids can reduce triglyceride levels, decrease the risk of heart arrhythmia (a leading cause of sudden death), decrease the amount of artery-clogging plaque, reduce unwanted blood clotting, improve the elasticity of arteries (prevents them from hardening), and even lowers blood pressure.

Natural Anti-inflammatory

Inflammation is the result of hormonal signals secreted by damaged bodily tissues triggered by an infection or injury. It perks up the immune system and causes swelling, tissue growth, and blood clotting. It is a good thing if it helps us heal from an injury such as a cut, but if unwanted, it can contribute to numerous health problems, from heart disease to arthritis to cancer to premature aging.

When the immune system senses an invading organism or an injury, it sends out white blood cells to clean up the problem. White blood cells, in turn, produce free radicals to kill any unwanted invaders and prevent the spread of infection, but sometimes the immune system goes overboard and doesn't know when to stop. Inflammation doesn't always stay localized in one area of the body; it can spread fairly quickly, damaging healthy cells and promoting the formation of yet more free radicals. An inflamed artery can cause a heart attack. An inflamed brain cell may be more vulnerable to Alzheimer's disease. An inflamed joint will become an arthritic joint.

Omega-3 fatty acids are your best defense against out-of-control inflammation. They reduce inflammation in the body, and can relieve the swelling and stiffness typical of inflammatory conditions such as rheumatoid arthritis. Even if you don't have arthritis, reducing inflammation can reduce your risk of nearly every degenerative disease.

Reduces the Risk of Cancer

There is compelling evidence that omega-3 fatty acids may protect against different types of cancer, particularly those that are hormone-sensitive. Notably, omega-3 fatty acids can inhibit the growth of breast, colon, pancreatic, and prostate tumors in animal and human cell studies. There is also a link between high intake of omega-3 fatty acids in the diet, notably from fish, and a lower risk of breast cancer, whereas a high intake of omega-6 fatty acids in the diet has been shown to increase the risk of developing certain types of cancer. I'm not suggesting that omega-3 fatty acids can totally prevent cancer, or cure it, but these good fats do offer some protection against cancer.

Eating the right kind of fat is fundamental to the Rosedale Diet, but so is eating the right kind of carbohydrates and protein. In the next chapter, I explain how to choose the right foods so that you can quickly shed excess pounds, trim the fat off your body, and enjoy optimal health.

chapter six

The Rosedale Diet Guide to Healthy Eating

O n the Rosedale Diet, you will be eating very differently than you have in the past. You will be adding new foods to your diet and eliminating other foods that are harmful to your health. Yet you will feel more satisfied and happier than you ever have felt on any other weight-loss program. For the first time, YOU will be in control of the hormones that have driven you to overeat and made you crave the wrong foods, not the other way around. You will no longer dread each meal as a test of your willpower. You will feel joyful again about eating because you are filling your plate with food that is making your body well toned and sleek, not fat and flabby. Not to mention the fact that you will be eating delicious food! Fat is the most flavorful part of any meal, and my good fat diet is packed with flavor. Read over the recipe list beginning on page 211. You will see an amazing selection of dishes to suit most any palate. You can snack on treats such as macadamia nuts and guacamole, forbidden foods on many other diets. There are even recipes for Shepherd's pie and pizza! And with each mouthful, you are protecting yourself against the degenerative diseases of aging and increasing the odds that you will live a longer, healthier life. What's not to like?

In the pages that follow, I explain everything you need to know about the meal plan so that you can succeed. Once you are familiar with the meal plan, you will see how easy it is to follow. To give you an idea of how to put meals together, starting on page 118, I provide four weeks of sample menus. You will find recipes in the Resources section starting on page 201. I'm providing these menus as guidelines, not to be rigidly followed. Once you learn my guidelines, you will be able to design your own meals, and even develop your own recipes, as do many of my patients.

▪ FOOD CHOICES: WHAT'S OPTIMAL?

Despite the zillions of products on supermarket shelves, nutrition comes down to five basic food groups: proteins, fats, carbohydrates, alcohol, and water. There's not too much controversy about water and alcohol; drink lots of clean water and you may drink up to one glass (4 ounces) of red wine daily. The real debate is over how much protein, fat, and carbs you should put on your plate to create the "optimal" diet. High carbohydrate–low fat diets have been the rage for decades (as we have become progressively fatter and more diabetic). More recently, low carbohydrate–high protein diets have become the latest trend. The problem is, neither is optimal. There is another possible combination that has been all but totally ignored—the Rosedale Diet, a high fat, low nonfiber carbohydrate, moderate protein diet. This is the *only* diet that will turn your cells into the most proficient fat burners and rid your body of the excess fat once and for all.

We humans eat for several reasons: For many of us, eating is as much a social activity as it is a biological imperative. We use mealtime as an opportunity to sit around the dining-room table and catch up with family and friends. Our holiday celebrations are often centered around a special meal. We use food as an escape from boredom or as a "treat." As food has taken on many different roles in society, however, we've lost touch with why we have to eat in the first place. As far as nature is concerned, we *must* eat for only two reasons: to obtain essential nutrients—vitamins, minerals, essential amino acids (from protein), and essential fatty acids (from good fat) that we cannot make ourselves and therefore must take in from our diet—to make new cells and repair old cells, and second, to obtain fuel so that our cells can do their jobs. Our cells burn either sugar or fat, which we get from food. Note: There are no carbohydrates on the list of essential nutrients. All carbohydrates are nonessential nutrients, that is, we don't need to eat them. Although our bodies do require some sugar, we can make all the sugar that we need from other nutrients. That means that you could be perfectly healthy if you never had an ounce of carbohydrate in your entire life!

■ CARBOHYDRATE: FIBER VS. NONFIBER

Carbohydrate refers to a vast category of food, including vegetables, fruits, all grains, pasta, bread, cereals, rice, potatoes, candy, cake, soda, and juice. All carbohydrates, however, are not equal. Carbohydrates have traditionally been classified as simple or complex, which has come to mean that simple are bad and complex are good. That classification is archaic and misleading, and ignores the last quarter-century of science. As I've said in previous chapters, most so-called complex carbohydrates turn to the simple sugar glucose within minutes after being eaten. Many of you are familiar with the glycemic index, a table that shows how fast foods turn into sugar after consumption. If you refer to the glycemic index, you will see that all complex carbohydrates including brown and wild rice, potatoes, cereals, pastas, and even "whole grain" bread turn to pure glucose shortly after being eaten. The glycemic index has become a popular tool to determine what to eat when following low carbohydrate diets. I believe it is useful as a tool to show the equivalency of complex carbohydrates and simple sugars, but it is not without drawbacks. First, it only measures glucose, and therefore the detrimental effects of other dangerous sugars such as fructose are hidden (see "Hidden Sources of Sugar" on page 80). Furthermore, for time and monetary constraints, the majority of experiments to determine the impact of a particular food on blood glucose is carried out for only three hours, and therefore the full impact of more slowly digestible carbohydrates is not measured. In many cases, the glycemic index tells only half the story and that is why I don't totally rely on it.

A more useful classification of carbohydrates is as either fiber or nonfiber carbohydrates. High fiber carbohydrates are found mostly in vegetables and nuts. The major advantage of fiber is that it can't be broken down into sugar, which means that it doesn't raise blood sugar levels or send your insulin and leptin levels soaring. In fact, only bacteria (including some that inhabit our gut) can digest fiber at all, and they digest a type of fiber called soluble fiber into good fats that are used for energy by the cells that line our intestines. (Having high quantities of these beneficial fats made by bacteria from fiber may be protective against colon cancer.) High fiber foods such as vegetables also fill you up, and can help control hunger (although restoring leptin sensitivity is the best way to control hunger!).

Any nonfiber carbohydrate that you eat can turn into some type of sugar and that sugar will be bad for you. It will combine with other vital molecular components (in a process called glycation) and prevent them from working properly by making them "sticky" and changing their shape. I've stated previously that nonfiber carbohydrates create a huge surge in both leptin and insulin. These foods will ultimately make you leptin resistant, fat, and sick. Remember, a bowl of cereal is a bowl of sugar, a slice of bread (with few exceptions) is a slice of sugar, and a potato is a big lump of sugar. Unfortunately, these are the foods that have become the mainstay of the American diet.

■ GRAINS

Although some grains contain a fair amount of fiber, they can also be converted into lots of sugar, and you should avoid them as much as possible. *Specifically, do not eat them at all the first three weeks you are on the Rosedale Diet meal plan with the exception of the few very high fiber-low sugar–producing grain products that I recommend on page 108.* I'm often asked, aren't grains necessary for health? Absolutely not! Grains were introduced late into the human diet—around 10,000 years ago—

and our ancestors survived millions of years without them. In modern times, grains have taken over supermarket shelves primarily because they are inexpensive to manufacture, ship, and store, whereas fresh vegetables can't be kept forever; they turn rotten within a relatively short period of time. Fresh fish is even more a problem in terms of a limited shelf life. There is a tremendous commercial incentive to stock stores with processed grain products over food with shorter shelf life.

We eat grains because we have become used to them and have learned to like them, not because we *need* them. I have enjoyed a nice, crusty piece of bread as much as the next person, but the fact is, I have learned not to miss carbs. I promise you that on the Rosedale Diet, you will not miss these foods as much, and you will learn to relish new foods. Furthermore, eating grains every day is definitely not worth the potential long-term health problems. Nonfiber carbs are highly addictive for many people, and a major source of sugar in the diet. I know you've been taught to think that whole wheat bread and whole grains such as millet, barley, oats, and rice are good for you. The fact is, you will be better off if you eliminate them as much as possible from your diet. Any starchy or sugary carbohydrate is going to send your leptin and insulin levels soaring, and over time, is going to create the metabolic hormonal roller coaster in your body that is the root cause of your food cravings and addictions. If you want to regain control of your weight, your health and ultimately your life, you need to get most grains off your plate. After you become a better fat burner, you can eat small amounts of grain in the form of a high fiber bread, a high fiber tortilla, and a high fiber cracker. (If you find that eating these foods makes you want more of them, don't eat them. If you are diabetic, you should avoid all sweets and starches. Period.)

■ NONSTARCHY VEGETABLES—THE BEST CARBS

Pile your plate high with nonstarchy vegetables. There are a great many of them to choose from, as you will see on page 107. (Exceptions include corn, beets, and lots of carrots—more than a few slices in your salad—which are very high in sugar, and should be avoided.) Not only are nonstarchy vegetables high in fiber, but their color pigments are beneficial. These pigments absorb radiation, which is why they have color, and are a natural source of antioxidants that can help control free radical damage in the body. I know that some of you may not like vegetables, or may think of them more as medicine than food. But your perceptions of food and flavors will change, I promise, and you will learn to like, if not love, your veggies. And as you regain leptin sensitivity, and your taste buds spring back to life, you will regain a new appreciation for the natural sweetness of vegetables like red peppers, snow peas, turnips, and cauliflower. And the starchy, sugary foods that you used to love will have an "off" taste.

Another benefit of vegetables is that they have lots of fiber, and fiber will fill you up. There are two ways that you feel like you've had enough to eat. The first is to feel like you are no longer hungry (satiated), which is what will happen when you are leptin sensitive. The second way is to fill your stomach with food, which is not as good, especially if you reach for the wrong foods. If you feel compelled to keep on eating, then reach for some high fiber vegetables and drink lots of water, which will create a feeling of fullness.

The standard American diet is lacking in vegetables, in contrast to other cuisines. Undoubtedly, you've heard a great deal about the Mediterranean diet, and the fact that people who live in Italy and Greece have much lower levels of heart disease and cancer than those in the United States. As mentioned earlier, people who follow the classic Mediterranean diet eat much more "good fat" than those eating the traditional Western diet, but they also eat many more servings of vegetables daily. They will routinely eat two to three different vegetables at each meal. Many Americans barely eat even one serving of vegetables daily with the exception of French fries!

▪ FRUIT

Fruit contains some fiber, which is fine, but it is also high in fructose, a type of sugar that is very harmful, as I will explain below in "Hidden Sources of Sugar." Fructose can also cause digestive problems, including gas, bloating, and diarrhea, which is why it's not a great idea to gorge on fruit. In my experience, I have found that once people cut out other sweets (cakes, cookies, candy) from their diet, they may compensate by overeating fruit when they crave sweets. Using fruit as a crutch won't help you overcome your need for sweets. Once you eliminate sugary foods from your diet, your taste buds will adjust to eating food that is not supersweet, and will actually begin to appreciate the natural flavor of food.

The best part of any fruit is in the skin because it contains the greatest amount of antioxidants to protect the inside of the fruit and seeds from radiation from the sun and from free radicals. Berries contain very high amounts of antioxidants in their skin, and are a great source of fiber. As far as I'm concerned, berries are the best fruit and the only fruit you should eat. Of all berries, blueberries are the best. I do allow some other fruits in limited amounts after the first few weeks of the program. There are some fruits, however, that are very high in sugar, and I prefer that you avoid them altogether (see page 117). The reality is, you don't need fruit to be healthy. You can get the same antioxidant boost from vegetables, but without the sugar, and often more fiber.

■ HIDDEN SOURCES OF SUGAR

When you think of sugar, you tend to think of the "obvious suspects"— the table sugar you use in your coffee, candy, soda, or desserts. The reality is, if you eat most prepared food (snack foods, frozen TV dinners, canned soup, packaged cereals, bread, frozen waffles, crackers, tomato sauce, condiments such as ketchup and steak sauce) you are eating sugar. Once you start reading food labels, you will be amazed to see that various forms of sugar (sucrose, corn syrup, high fructose corn syrup, dextrose, turbinado, maple sugar, etc.) are common ingredients in prepared food. Organic, so-called "natural" sugar or honey is no better. Some experts estimate that many people may unknowingly be eating between forty to sixty teaspoons of sugar a day in their food. I tell my patients to avoid products with added sugar.

I am particularly worried about the high rate of consumption of high fructose corn syrup, or fructose, a cheap, very sweet sugar which is finding its way into more and more prepared foods. Although fructose is low on the glycemic index (it does not convert easily to glucose), it can cause serious health problems, the primary ones being that it promotes insulin resistance and fat storage. It actually causes more damage inside your body than glucose, which is found in table sugar (a combination of fructose and glucose). Researchers have routinely fed laboratory mice fructose to induce insulin resistant diabetes to test antidiabetic drugs! I urge you to be especially vigilant about avoiding foods high in fructose or high fructose syrup.

▪ ARTIFICIAL SWEETENERS

I don't recommend that people use a lot of artificial sweeteners, including aspartame, sucralose, or saccharin. They are loaded with chemicals, and I don't think you should eat artificial foods. Moreover, they simply perpetuate sweet cravings and desensitize your sweet receptors. It's far better to increase your sweet sensitivity to the natural sweet taste of foods than to load up on fake sugar.

Stevia (from the stevia leaf) is a noncaloric sweetener sold at natural food stores. It's not artificial, nor is it as sweet as table sugar. It is used as a sugar substitute in the Raspberry Mousse Cake recipe on page 285 because it's far better than sugar, but I strongly caution against eating too many sweets that can trigger starch and sugar cravings.

▪ PROTEIN

Protein is an essential nutrient—you can't live without it. Protein is broken down by digestion into amino acids, which provide the building blocks for structure and repair for the body. Amino acids form muscle, make enzymes, and repair and make new cells. Everything that is transcribed by your genes is a protein enzyme! Without protein, your body would not be able to function. If you don't get enough protein from your diet, your body will rob it from your lean mass (muscle and bone) which will make you weak and frail before your time.

The fact that protein is essential for life, however, doesn't mean that you can eat it in unlimited quantities. When you eat more protein than your body needs to replace and repair body parts, excess protein is largely converted into glucose and burned as fuel. It turns you into a sugar maker and sugar burner! This is not desirable or healthy. On the Rosedale Diet, I limit the amount of protein that you can eat daily. I advise most people to eat between 50 and 75 grams of protein daily (depending on their body size, height, frame, and activity level), spread out among their meals with not more than 15–20 grams per meal. (See charts beginning on page 207 to calculate the right amount of protein for you.) That's enough protein for the body to do its work, but not so much so that you will burn it as fuel, which will prevent you from burning off excess fat as fuel.

Most of your protein should come from fish and (skinless) poultry which is low in saturated and omega-6 fats, and to a lesser extent from foods that contain more saturated fat, such as beef. Nonfat or low fat dairy products (in limited quantities) are another acceptable source of protein. You will also get some protein from eating nuts and eggs.

I know that many popular diets today allow you to eat all the protein you want, to lose weight, as long as you avoid most carbohydrates. On the surface, this is a very appealing promise. Many of these diets lump all protein sources together, and allow you to gorge on high saturated fat cuts of meat such as rib steaks and brisket, and even cured meats such as pastrami and hot dogs as long as you stay away from carbs. And at least initially, most people lose weight. However, our goal is not just to lose weight, but to lose *fat* and achieve maximal health. If you cut carbs out of your diet and load up on protein, you will lose some weight, no question about it. But high protein–low carbohydrate diets, like other diets, are not long-term solutions. I have treated hundreds of patients who have been on such diets, but who have reached a plateau with still more fat to lose, and they are not healthy. Many still have carbohydrate cravings! Why? Because the extra protein they are eating is being converted into glucose and burned as sugar, which causes spikes

Avoid eating a protein-laden meal late at night. Burning protein will rev up your metabolism and heat you up, just at a time when you want your body to be cooling off and winding down for sleep.

in leptin and insulin levels, which in turn cause sugar cravings. These diets are particularly bad for diabetic patients because they can raise blood sugar and insulin levels.

There are other reasons why a high protein diet falls short of the ideal diet. As you know by now, the type of fat you eat is very important. Foods high in protein are generally high in saturated fat. Saturated fat is much harder to burn off than good fat (until you become a good fat burner), so if you eat high amounts of saturated fat, you will interfere with your body's ability to burn fat. A diet high in saturated fat promotes insulin resistance, and may increase the risk of heart disease. To me, the goal is not about weight loss. It is to achieve optimal health and to lose undesirable weight as a result.

To compound the problem, a diet heavy in protein can produce toxic by-products. A protein molecule consists of an amino (nitrogen) group attached to a carbon chain. To metabolize almost any amino acid to use as fuel, you must first deaminate or remove the nitrogen group. Your body can recycle some of the nitrogen to make nonessential amino acids, or you must dispose of the nitrogen by making the toxic by-products of ammonia and urea that can overburden your kidneys. The more protein that you eat, the more toxic waste you must spend considerable energy getting rid of. That energy could otherwise have been used more appropriately to maintain and repair yourself—to become healthier, slow aging, and live longer.

Perhaps the worst part about eating excess protein is often touted as one of its benefits: Protein is the most thermogenic food and as I discussed in Chapter 4, creating excess heat is harmful to your body.

Finally, a high protein diet does not restore leptin sensitivity as well as my regimen, which is key to permanent fat loss and optimal health.

The Rosedale Diet meal plan restores leptin sensitivity better than any other popular diet, and in fact is the only diet that I know of (other than severe caloric restriction) that has ever been able to show a restoration of leptin sensitivity.

■ FISH

Fish is a great source of both good fat and protein. Some types of fish (sardines, salmon, tuna, mackerel, herring, trout, orange roughy, halibut) are high in beneficial omega-3 fatty acids, and I highly recommend them. Most other types of fish are also fine (for a complete list of recommended fish, turn to page 105). It doesn't matter whether fish is fresh, canned, or "fresh" frozen fish; the fat content remains the same. Try to buy wild rather than farm-raised fish. (Ask at the fish counter whether or not the fish is wild or farm-raised. You are more likely to find wild fish at health food stores or fish markets.) Farmed fish are typically raised in unnatural conditions, and may be given antibiotics to prevent disease, and growth hormone and other chemicals to stimulate growth. Fish shouldn't be loaded up with chemicals, and neither should you! There is one exception to the no-farmed fish rule: A small number of organic fish farms have sprung up in Europe and the United States that do not use hormones, antibiotics or other chemicals, and do not use grain feed (which is not what fish eat under normal circumstances!). Organically raised fish may be found at some natural foods supermarkets, gourmet shops, and even discount stores. I found an organically raised smoked salmon sold at Costco (their own house brand) that was quite good and easy on the pocketbook.

If you use fresh fish, be sure to buy the freshest fish from a reputable fish market, natural foods store, or supermarket. If you buy a whole fish, make sure that the eyes are bright, and not cloudy. Truly fresh fish does not have a strong "fishy" odor.

If you can't get to the fish market to buy fresh fish, keeps of cans of sardines (in olive oil), salmon, tuna (dolphin-free, please), and shrimp in your pantry for a quick meal.

THE BENEFITS OF EATING THE RIGHT AMOUNT OF PROTEIN . . . AND NOT TOO MUCH

- Increases fat burning. Eating more protein than you need reduces your ability to burn fat.
- Reduces blood sugar. Eating extra protein causes you to turn protein, including some of your muscle and bone, into sugar.
- Enhances insulin (and leptin) sensitivity. This helps everybody and especially those with metabolic "diseases," including diabetes, heart and vascular disease, and obesity.
- Reduces risk of a heart attack.
- Keeps you running "cool" and efficient. Extra protein creates lots of extra heat.
- Reduces free radical damage and increases important antioxidants in your cells.
- Reduces the rate of aging, enhancing your health and life span.

As good as fish is, it is not a problem-free food. Due to water pollution, some fish is contaminated with mercury, a neurotoxin that is particularly dangerous to the brain. To my way of thinking, the small amount of mercury you may get from eating fish does not negate the positive health benefits of most fish. It's good common sense to avoid eating fish that have the highest levels of mercury; these include shark, swordfish, king mackerel, and tile fish. Pregnant women need to be especially careful to avoid fish high in mercury because of potential harm to the fetus. If you are very concerned about mercury, stick to fish that are lowest in mercury content, such as fresh, wild Pacific or Alaskan salmon and sardines (which are also terrific sources of omega-3 fatty acids), tilapia, and haddock. But don't stop eating fish!

I am frequently asked this question on talk shows: If I had only one food to take with me to a deserted island, which food would it be. Without missing a beat, I always answer sardines packed in olive oil. They are high in good oils including omega-3 and (omega-9) monounsaturated fats, a good source of protein, and contain almost no carbohydrate. Sardines are also generally very low in toxic metals.

Not everyone likes fish, but everyone needs the good fat in fish. Cod liver oil is a fine substitute for the real thing (I prefer bottled oil as opposed to gelcaps). The brand I recommend (Carlson Norweigan Cod Liver Oil) has a pleasant, lemony flavor that can be tolerated by even the most ardent fish haters. It also is filtered of all detectable traces of mercury and other toxic metals.

A note to sushi lovers: Sushi is fine as long as you eat the fish and not the rice (just order the sashimi). If you eat sushi, be sure it's from a reputable restaurant that uses only the freshest fish.

■ BEEF, LAMB, AND PORK

If you're trying to become a proficient fat burner, I recommend that you eliminate all beef, lamb, and pork from your diet, at least for the first three weeks you are on the meal plan (unless it is not grain-fed). Even the leanest cuts of meat have a fair amount of saturated fat, which is precisely the fat you're trying to lose. It doesn't make much sense to eat what you're trying to get rid of. Once you become a more proficient fat burner, you can add meat back to your diet as long as you stick to the leanest cuts.

The degree of saturated fat in meat varies widely depending on the cut. Please choose your meat selections from the foods listed in "B" Proteins. Don't eat more than two meat meals a week. If you do happen to slip up and eat a fatty cut of meat (for example, prime rib, which is high in saturated fat, is often served at weddings or parties), do some exercise afterward to burn it off. Some cuts of pork can be almost pure fat, so avoid those that are not on the list of acceptable pork cuts. You will notice that I do not include any bacon or cured meats such as smoked sausage. Cured meats contain preservatives called nitrites, which are converted into nitrosamines, a very potent carcinogen in the colon. Some health food stores sell noncured bacon, which is preferable, but it tends to be high in saturated fat. Turkey bacon is another option, but it often contains lots of dyes and chemicals to make it look like the real thing, so I don't recommend it. This doesn't mean that you have nothing to team up with your eggs in the morning. Turkey sausage, which is sold at health food stores and most supermarkets, is a wonderful alternative to the real thing. Do read the food labels carefully to make sure that the sausage is preservative-free and doesn't contain a lot of additives. Regardless, don't overdo the protein. Don't eat more than two pieces of sausage and one egg in the same meal.

Not all beef is the same. Most cattle go to feed lots and are fed a diet of grain for several weeks to fatten them up, along with a dose of antibiotics to prevent infection, and some growth hormones to speed everything up. They get little or no exercise to make sure that they fatten up as quickly as possible. Like grain-fed people, grain-fed cattle make lots of saturated fat. That's why I said earlier that eating grain-fed beef is just another way of eating starchy carbohydrates—ultimately, it has nearly the same negative effects on your body. You get many of the disadvantages of grains (saturated fat) without the redeeming element of fiber. There is a healthier alternative to "feed lot" beef: naturally raised, and only grass-fed beef that has never been to a feed lot. Beef from cattle that have never been to a feed lot is relatively low in saturated fat, and higher in beneficial omega-3 fatty acids than grain-fed beef. Exclusively grass-fed beef looks and tastes the way beef used to taste—it has a mild, subtle flavor and is not dripping in grease. If you're used to high fat cuts of meat, switching to exclusively grass-fed beef may take some getting used to, but I promise, you will adapt to the new lighter taste and texture very quickly.

You can purchase grass-fed beef at some gourmet shops, natural supermarkets, or by mail order or on the Internet. (See list of grass-fed beef providers in "Rosedale Resources.") I recommend that all patients have their ferritin (stored iron) levels measured. Those people with high ferritin levels should not eat very much red meat until their ferritin level is brought down by donating blood. See page 188.

■ GAME MEATS

In recent years, game meats (such as buffalo and venison) have been growing in popularity, and have been popping up on menus in restaurants throughout the country. Game meats are high in protein and low in fat. They do not contain any hormones or antibiotics, and are a great alternative to beef. In some health conscious parts of the country (like in Denver where I live), buffalo burger is becoming almost as popular as regular hamburger!

■ EGGS

Just like beef, most chickens are raised in confinement, fed grains, and loaded with antibiotics and growth hormones. These chickens produce eggs that are relatively high in saturated fat and low in omega-3 fatty acids, not to mention what other chemical residue may find its way into both the chicken and the eggs. A better alternative to standard commercially produced eggs is to buy eggs from free-range chickens that are fed a special vegetarian diet of either flaxseed or algae. Not only are the chickens healthier on the diet, but their eggs contain a high amount of beneficial omega-3 fatty acids, which will make you healthier. There are several brands of omega-3 enriched eggs on the market, including Gold Circle Farms, the brand that I use. You can buy omega-3 enriched eggs at most health food stores and many supermarkets. They are a bit more expensive than regular eggs, but the nutritional benefits are well worth the difference.

■ POULTRY

Try to use organic poultry that is hormone-free and antibiotic-free. At one time, it was difficult finding organic poultry; today however, it is sold in most health food stores and many supermarkets.

Although free-range poultry is raised in a healthier environment than caged animals, please handle it with care in your kitchen. All poultry can be tainted with salmonella, a bacterium that is a major cause of food poisoning in humans. Cooking poultry thoroughly (until the juices are clear) will kill the germs that cause salmonella poisoning. It's important to remember to wash any cutting boards, countertops, or implements that come in contact with poultry (or meat) very carefully with hot water and soap.

■ DAIRY

Most dairy products are loaded with saturated fat, and I don't recommend many of them. I do allow (in limited quantities) low fat cottage cheese, low fat cream cheese, low fat ricotta cheese, and Jarlsberg Lite Swiss cheese. Once again, if you have a choice, purchase organic products from cows raised without hormones or other chemicals.

I don't believe that anyone should drink cow's milk—and that goes for kids, too. Humans are the only species on the planet that drink milk after weaning and it is not necessary or even healthy. Full fat milk (and even 2 percent) is very high in saturated fat. Milk is also loaded with a sugar called lactose, known for causing digestive problems in many people (so-called lactose intolerance). Lactose is made up of the sugars glucose and galactose, another very unhealthy and dangerous sugar. Milk also contains casein, a protein to which many people are allergic and that has been implicated in the kind of autoimmune reactions that can lead to type 1 diabetes. Several studies have found that infants who are fed cow's milk are more likely to develop diabetes than those who are breast-fed. As a physician who treats diabetes and sees the awful health consequences of this disease, I am horrified at the thought that so many of my colleagues are recommending that children eat a food that can cause them long-term harm. I'm frequently asked, if they don't drink milk, where will children get calcium for strong teeth and bones? Despite all the hype about milk and the importance of calcium supplements to strong bones, only rarely does a deficiency of milk or dietary calcium in this country have anything to do with the cause of osteoporosis, and I defy anyone to show me a convincing study that says otherwise. Think about it. Other large mammals, such as lions, tigers, and bears have very strong teeth and bones without drinking a drop of milk after weaning. Of course, we need some calcium in our diet, but we humans can get all the calcium we need from nuts, green leafy vegetables, and sardine bones. We don't need or even want that much of it if we use calcium efficiently.

You may be surprised to learn that it is mostly the protein content in bones that make them strong, not so much the amount of calcium they contain. If your cells are insulin and leptin resistant, and you are constantly being forced to burn sugar, your body will begin to chew up the protein in your bone to burn as fuel, and it doesn't matter if you are drinking a quart of milk a day or gobbling down calcium supplements. When it comes to calcium, it's not so much the quantity that matters, but the quality of instructions that tell your body what to do with it. Once again, those pivotal instructions of where to put the calcium come from leptin. If you're leptin resistant, your cells are likely to "misplace" calcium, that is, it is more likely to end up in your arteries (where it can cause a heart attack) than in your bones. Bottom line: You should not drink milk, and you don't need to take calcium supplements.

■ LEGUMES

With the exception of black soybeans, most legumes are not a great source of protein and are high in carbohydrate. (Black soybeans are a type of soybean that is especially high in fiber and protein, and are sold in bulk or cooked in cans at health food stores and many supermarkets.) Stick to small beans (the more skin, the more fiber) and limit your intake of legumes to no more than three meals a week. (For a list of acceptable legumes, see page 108.) If you are diabetic or have heart or vascular disease, you should avoid most legumes.

I do allow small amounts of hummus (made out of chickpeas) on the meal plan. Hummus also contains olive oil and garlic, which helps offset some of the bad carbohydrates. Nevertheless, I don't want you to gorge on it; use it sparingly as a condiment.

▪ HOW TO GET GOOD FAT IN YOUR DIET

Nuts

When the "all fat is bad" craze took hold in the 1970s, nuts were all but eliminated from most of the popular no-fat diets. Rich in fat, nuts were dismissed as worthless by nutrition experts obsessed with cutting fat out of the diet at all costs. But it soon became apparent that this approach was, well, just plain nutty. Study after study began appearing in medical journals noting that people who eat nuts have a lower incidence of heart disease and are generally healthier than nonnut eaters. Grudgingly, even the most antinut fanatic had to concede that maybe there was something good in nuts. We now know that the "good" in nuts was mostly fat. Nuts are high in monounsaturated fat and give you energy without sending your leptin levels soaring. Nut critics are now eating their words. The FDA recently approved nuts for the first health claim to be used on package labels. The claim states, "Scientific evidence suggests but does not prove that eating 1.5 ounces per day of most nuts, as part of a diet low in saturated fat and cholesterol, may reduce the risk of heart disease."

I'm not certain whether monounsaturated fats themselves offer special health benefits, or whether nut eaters are healthier because of what they are not eating in their place, that is, high sugar foods or other bad fats. Frankly, it doesn't matter. Chock-full of good fats, nuts not only quell your hunger, but promote fat burning. The one caveat is, nuts will only promote fat burning as long you don't eat them with starchy or sugary foods.

On the Rosedale Diet, there is a wide variety of nuts to choose from (see list on page 103). Nuts make a great portable snack, and quench hunger pangs very quickly. When you are hungry, I recommend that you eat seven or eight nuts at a time (slowly, don't bolt them down) and you will be amazed how fast you will be satiated. (Cracking your own nuts can help prevent eating too many at one time.) If you're hungry forty-five minutes later, eat a few more! Nut butters are also great on vegetables or on low carb crackers. I prefer that you use the raw, unsalted nuts and nut butters that are sold in health stores, if possible, since heating nuts can promote oxidation.

If you look at the list of acceptable nuts, you will see one omission—PEANUTS. Peanuts are not nuts at all, they are legumes. I don't recommend that anyone eat them for three reasons: (1) They are highly allergenic, (2) they are prone to develop a carcinogenic mold called aflatoxin, and (3) they're high in omega-6 fatty acids and a poor source of monounsaturates and omega-3s.

A word about cashews. Although cashews are allowed on the Rosedale Diet, eat them sparingly because they have less fiber than other nuts and are higher in nonfiber carbs.

If you've never eaten a nut butter other than peanut butter, you're in for a real treat. Almond butter and cashew butter are lighter in texture and I think more flavorful than peanut butter. If you are allergic to peanuts, I recommend that you make your own nut butter at home. Commercial nut butters may be processed in the same plant with peanuts, which could cause cross-contamination.

About 1 percent of the population is allergic to tree nuts. If you are allergic to nuts, don't eat them, and substitute another acceptable food in place of your nut servings.

▪ WHAT TO DRINK?

Please drink eight to ten glasses of filtered or bottled water daily. That's right, WATER. Not fruit juice, regular soda, or diet soda. Stick to water or unsweetened herbal teas. If you must drink regular tea, drink decaf. If you love coffee, and are not too sick with diabetes, high blood pressure, or heart disease, a single cup of coffee (decaf preferred) is okay if that's what it takes to keep you on the program. Do try some coffee substitutes, such as Teeccino, which is sold at health food stores and some supermarkets. Many people find that they are perfectly acceptable alternatives to the real thing.

Better to drink before or after your meal. When you eat, your body produces digestive enzymes to help break down the food into its essential nutrients. If you flood your system with fluid while you are eating, you can interfere with this process. Elderly people especially should try to not drink too much water during their meal, since they may have insufficient acid or digestive enzymes that could get too diluted.

■ WHAT ABOUT ALCOHOL?

Alcohol is a double-edged sword. On the one hand, some studies show that a drink or two a day can reduce the risk of heart disease, but on the other, we know that alcohol inhibits fat burning. Moreover, alcohol can boost estrogen levels in women, and may increase the risk of breast cancer. I've given the alcohol issue a great deal of thought, and I've reached the conclusion that alcohol is probably helpful to people who are very stressed out, but by no means essential for health. Alcohol lowers blood pressure and has a relaxing effect on the body, which may be beneficial to people who have difficulty winding down. A better way to reduce stress, I believe, is to practice yoga or other stress-reduction techniques. Please keep in mind that more than one or two drinks daily has been shown to be harmful to your health. If you do drink, avoid sweet mixed drinks, and stick to red wine, low carb beer, or pure spirits. There are some new low carb beers on the market that are actually quite good and are a good compromise.

■ THE BEST WAY TO COOK YOUR FOOD

Vegetables

Vegetables can be eaten raw, steamed, or lightly sautéed. Cooking vegetables in a microwave oven can destroy B vitamins, including folic acid, which helps protect against both heart disease and cancer. Use the microwave only as a last resort. Don't douse your vegetables with butter or cream sauces if you are trying to lose weight. Try using olive, almond, or avocado oil.

Fish

Fish should be broiled, sautéed (only in good fat such as olive, avocado, or almond oil), baked, or poached in as little fat as possible. Smoked fish is fine, as long as you don't make a steady diet of it. (The smoking process can produce carcinogenic chemicals.) Do not fry fish! Don't smother fish in heavy butter or cream sauces that will only increase its saturated fat content, especially during the first three weeks of the diet.

Meat

Cooking meat—especially fatty meat—at very high temperatures (such as grilling) may increase the risk of stomach cancer. Heat produces carcinogenic compounds called heterocyclic aromatic amines (HAAs.) Partaking in the occasional barbecue probably isn't going to hurt you, but don't make it a habit. If you like to grill outdoors, stick to lean cuts of meat. It's also a good idea to partially cook the food indoors in your oven or microwave before placing it on the grill. This will reduce the amount of time the meat is being cooked over hot coals. Indoor grilling machines are a good alternative to outdoor grilling. On most indoor grills, the fat drips off the meat into a fat collector, reducing the amount of harmful chemicals produced in the cooking process. If you broil food in your oven, put the food in an unheated broiler to avoid cooking at excessively high temperatures. Baking, sautéeing, or poaching are healthier cooking methods.

Undercooked meat, especially hamburger, can be a breeding ground for E. coli bacteria. Even though I don't want you overheating your meat, that doesn't mean that it should not be thoroughly cooked.

Invest in a meat thermometer. It will help prevent overcooking. Cook beef steaks and roasts to a minimum internal temperature of 145 degrees F. Ground beef must be cooked to a minimum internal temperature of 160 degrees F.

Pork roasts and chops must be cooked to a minimum internal temperature of 155 degrees F., and ground pork should be cooked to 160 degrees F.

Cook lamb to a minimal internal temperature of 160 degrees F.

CAUTION: Cook all meat and poultry at temperatures above 325 degrees F.

Game Meats

Game meats should be cooked the same as beef. Since these meats tend to be very lean, you should marinate them for flavor and to retain moisture before cooking.

Poultry

Bake, sauté (in good fat), grill, or poach in little or no fat. Almost all commercially available poultry is grain-fed and therefore high in saturated fat. Most of the fat in poultry is in the skin, but removing the skin before cooking can make it dry. A good compromise is to keep the skin on during cooking, but to peel it off before you eat it. Whole chickens and Cornish game hens should be cooked to an internal temperature of 180 degrees F. (Stick the meat thermometer into the thigh to get an accurate reading.) Breasts with or without the bone should be cooked to 170 degrees F. Other parts, including the legs, thighs, and drumsticks, should be cooked to 180 degrees F. A whole turkey is done when the internal temperature reaches 180 degrees F. (Stick the thermometer into the drumstick to get an accurate reading.)

Eggs

The yolk of the egg is high in fat and very vulnerable to oxidation, especially so in high-omega-3 eggs, and especially if it is cooked at very high temperatures. Therefore, I do not recommend cooking methods for

HEY, DOC, WHAT SHOULD I EAT FOR BREAKFAST?

Patients frequently ask, "If I can't eat a bagel or cereal in the morning, what can I eat?" The fact is, humans are the only species on the planet to make a distinction between what they eat in the A.M. and in the P.M. I believe that this is due to constant bombardment by the food industry promoting cereal (pure sugar) as the ideal breakfast food. It's far preferable to start the day with a protein shake, a poached egg with turkey sausage, or even some chicken salad, as I often do.

eggs that produce excess heat (such as frying). Egg yolks should always be cooked *under water* where the temperature cannot exceed 212 degrees F., and where they are less likely to be exposed to oxygen. Eggs can be poached, soft-boiled, or slightly hard-boiled (not overcooked—the yolk can still be slightly firm, but not tough, and the outside of the yolk should not have turned green). If you crave an omelette, you can have one as long as you just use the egg whites, which have no fat to oxidize and will not be adversely affected by heat.

■ EATING ON THE RUN

Don't Leave Home Without Your Snacks! Carry a selection of healthy snacks with you wherever you go. Cut vegetables (with nut butter) and nuts are portable snacks that can go without refrigeration for the entire day. Carry a small, soft-sided cooler with you if necessary to keep perishable foods fresh.

Eating in most restaurants is not a problem, as long as you know what and how to order:

■ Skip the complementary bread or chips. No need to tempt yourself; simply ask the waiter to remove them from the table.

HOW MUCH PROTEIN SHOULD YOU EAT?

This is not a high protein diet; this is a diet in which you eat the optimal amount of protein to keep your body running well. Ideally, you should eat approximately between 60 and 75 grams of protein daily or three to five portions of protein daily (between 15 and 20 grams each). How do you know how much protein is right for you? It varies according to body size, frame, and activity level. A 5'3" woman with small bones will require less protein than a 6'4" man. (The smaller woman can eat about three protein portions daily while the bigger man can eat four to five.) If the woman is very physically active, she can eat a bit more protein (maybe one extra portion daily) than if she is sedentary. This isn't rocket science; all you need to do is make a good estimate of your protein needs, and try not to exceed them. You don't have to eat exactly the right amount of protein grams daily to succeed on my program, but you should try to stay as close to my guidelines as possible. (If you are diabetic, however, you must be very strict about protein consumption.)

There are people who do better having exact guidelines for their protein intake, and who will find that they "cheat" too much if they don't have hard and fast numbers to follow. If you are one of them, turn to page 205 for a more precise way of figuring out your protein daily allowance.

For the rest of you, here's an easy to way to keep track of your protein portions for the day without carrying around a food scale.

Your major sources of protein are meat, fish, poultry, eggs, and dairy products.

- One portion of meat, fish, or poultry is equal in size to about one deck of cards and contains 15 grams of protein.
- One portion of soft cheese (low fat cottage cheese or ricotta cheese) is equal in size to ½ cup and contains 14 grams of protein.
- Two eggs contain 14 grams of protein.
- One protein shake contains about 15 grams of protein (or about ⅔ of a scoop).

A word of caution. Read food labels. Some products (such as low carb bread or tortilla wrap) may contain up to 9 grams of protein per serving, and should be included in your daily protein count.

- Go right to reading the fish or poultry dishes on the menu. If possible, choose the ones that contain the right kinds of oil (salmon, tuna, mackerel, herring, trout, orange roughy, and halibut). Be sure to ask that your meal be prepared using olive oil rather than other vegetable oils or margarine, or simply broiled with lemon. Butter is acceptable for cooking in small quantities. In Chinese restaurants, ask for the food to be cooked in a wok in water rather than vegetable oil.
- If your entrée comes with a starch, request extra grilled vegetables instead or an extra salad.
- If you are in a diner, you can always order a poached egg with turkey sausage (without toast or potatoes).
- Many restaurants today offer grilled chicken or fish over greens. Chicken Caesar or blackened chicken or shrimp salad is fine, as long as you tell the waiter to hold the croutons and the salad dressing. Dress your salad with vinaigrette or olive oil and vinegar. If you are in an Asian restaurant, order steamed vegetables with chicken or fish served without a heavy sauce. Ask your waiter not to bring rice with your meal.
- Order water, decaffeinated or herbal tea with your meal.
- Fast-food restaurants where you have little control over how food is cooked, and the kind of oils used in cooking, are not the best choice.
- Most major cities have natural food restaurants where you can get fresh, organic food cooked simply to your specifications.

■ ROSEDALE'S RULES

FEEL GOOD ABOUT YOURSELF. You are about to embark on a program that will produce wonderful results for your body. You will learn a new way of eating that will make you look better and feel better than you have in years. Within a short time—usually within two to three weeks—most of you will notice that you look leaner, your clothes fit better, and you have energy to spare. There will also be some amazing things happening to you that aren't visible, yet are more important. Your Longevity Profile—that is, your biomarkers of aging—will be vastly improved as you regain your leptin sensitivity, and along with losing excess fat you will be de-aging your body and reinventing your body. So smile, feel good about taking this positive step, and get started.

AVOID SUGAR AND STARCH. To jump-start the fat burning process, during the first three weeks on the meal plan, eat as little non-fiber starch or sugar as possible. You don't have to count carb grams; just don't eat nonfiber carbs. Avoid all starches such as potatoes, bread, rice, pasta, potatoes, cereal, corn, and ALL GRAINS (yes, even whole grains). Fill up with your plate with vegetables, with the exception of those high in sugar, including beets, yams, carrots, or tomatoes (though a few sliced carrots or cherry tomatoes in salads is okay). Limit your fruit intake to a small amount (¼ cup maximum daily) of berries, preferably blueberries. (Diabetics should avoid starch and sugar all the time.) After the first three weeks, you can add a bit more starch to your diet (such as a couple of slices of high fiber, low carb bread), as long as this does not increase your cravings for more.

DON'T BE AFRAID OF FAT—BUT EAT GOOD FAT. This is a high fat diet—EAT FAT IF YOU ARE HUNGRY! But stick to the good fats found in nuts, avocados, fatty fish, olives, etc.

LIMIT SATURATED FAT FOR THE FIRST THREE WEEKS. When you want to lose weight, what you really want to lose is *saturated fat*. So stop eating it, at least for the first three weeks you are on the meal plan. Pass on the beef, pork, lamb, and most dairy products and eat primarily fish, nuts, chicken, vegetables, and no-fat cheese. After the first three weeks on the meal plan, you can eat foods that are higher in saturated fat (such as lean beef, lamb, and pork), although those wishing to continue losing weight should not eat very much of these foods.

EAT THE RIGHT AMOUNT OF PROTEIN FOR YOU. Remember, this is a high fat diet, not a high protein diet. You should eat the right amount of protein for your body type.

EAT WHEN YOU ARE HUNGRY. I don't want you to walk around hungry. When you are hungry, eat good fats, protein (if you have not exceeded your protein limit), and fiber (like vegetables). Good snacks include raw or dry roasted nuts, nut butters, guacamole, and vegetables and dip. (See Recipes section beginning on page 211.) You should not be hungry on this diet. I mean it! If you are hungry, have a few nuts or any of the healthy snacks listed in the menus. If you have trouble feeling full without eating a lot of starch, fill up on vegetables. Your cravings for sweets and starches, which are similar to an addiction, should subside within three weeks.

DRINK LOTS OF WATER. Stick to water, seltzer, or flavored water (tea and herbal teas). No soda of any type, even diet soda, and no juice.

DON'T EAT A LOT AT ONE TIME. When you are hungry, eat a small meal or snack. It's far better for your metabolism to eat several small meals or snacks throughout the day than three large meals.

EAT SLOWLY. If you bolt down your food, your brain will not have the chance to know that you should no longer be hungry, and you will keep eating. If you eat slowly, your brain will get the message that you are filling up, and you will know when it's time to stop eating.

DON'T EAT FOR AT LEAST THREE HOURS BEFORE BED-TIME. Your last meal in the evening should be at least twelve hours from your first meal of the morning. This will give your body the time it needs to rest and heal, and you will find that you are sleeping better. Digesting food is hard work. Let your digestive system sleep also. Drinking water, however, is okay.

EXERCISE AFTER THE LAST MEAL OF THE DAY (IF POS-SIBLE). Do fifteen to twenty minutes of mild resistance exercise (see Chapter 9) or take a short walk (preferably uphill). This will help burn up sugar, and prime you for a night of fat burning. Then you should keep burning fat all night long, and the more fat you burn, the better you get at it. Even broccoli has some sugar and I want you to burn it off as soon as possible. What I don't want you to do is to eat late, lie down on the sofa and go to sleep. This will force your body to be working hard trying to digest all that food just when it should be winding down for sleep.

And finally . . .

DON'T SLIP UP—AT LEAST FOR THE FIRST THREE

WEEKS. It takes about three weeks for your metabolism to retool so that you switch from being a "sugar burner" to a "fat burner." Once your body and brain have made the switch, you will feel the difference. You will have more energy, better mental focus, and you'll even be sleeping better! In my experience, I have found that after feeling the difference, and "retooling" the brain's needs and desires, few people want to go back to their old eating patterns.

NOBODY'S PERFECT. It is far better not to, but IF YOU DO SLIP UP . . . EXERCISE IT OFF. If you "forget" and eat a sandwich with two slices of bread, or eat a cookie, go for a brisk twenty- to thirty-minute walk or undertake other exercise immediately after eating. If you don't burn off those starchy calories right away, they will raise your blood sugar, raise your leptin and insulin levels, prevent fat burning, and turn to fat, all of which get you right back to a deranged metabolism.

chapter seven

Getting Started: Weeks One to Three

The Rosedale Diet is divided into two levels: Level 1 and Level 2. I consider Level 1 to be the healthiest possible diet, and one that will not only help you lose weight quickly, but will give you the best shot at longevity. You must stay on Level 1 for at least three weeks, but some of you may opt to stay on it indefinitely. It is basically the diet that I follow most of the time.

Level 2 contains a wider variety of foods (a few more servings of fruit and starches) but it is still a very healthy diet.

You will make your food choices from the food lists starting on page 103.

The Rosedale Diet food lists are divided into three categories:

- A. The "A" list contains the best possible food choices. Plan most of your menus around these foods. While you are on Level 1, for the first three weeks on the Rosedale Diet, only eat foods on the "A" list.
- B. The "B" list contains foods that you can eat on an occasional basis when you are in Level 2, after the first three weeks you are on the diet. If you have a

metabolic problem such as insulin resistance or diabetes, or if you want to achieve optimal results in terms of weight loss and longevity, I recommend that you stick to the "A" list as much as possible.

■ C. The "C" list contains foods that you should avoid, and will only sabotage your efforts to regain leptin sensitivity and achieve permanent weight loss. DON'T EAT THEM!

■ SNACK WHENEVER YOU ARE HUNGRY. (Check out the sample meal plans on pages for suggestions of acceptable snacks.)

■ KEEP A FOOD DIARY

Learning a new way of eating can be a challenge, and it is very easy to lose track of your meals. To make it simple, I recommend that you keep a food diary for the first three weeks you are on the Rosedale Diet. Write down everything you eat—including snacks and beverages. To make it easy for you, you can use the Food Diary on page 203 in the "Rosedale Resources" section to keep track of your meals and snacks. In addition, you should keep track of the amount of protein that you are eating. I have found that when patients reduce their intake of carbohydrates, they often overconsume protein, and underconsume good fats.

■ THE "A" LIST:

PLAN MOST OF YOUR MEALS AND SNACKS FROM THIS LIST

"A" List Fat Sources

NUTS AND NUT BUTTERS (*eat in limited quantities)

Preferably raw, unroasted, and unsalted.
Nuts are also a good source of protein.

Almonds
Brazil nuts
Cashews*
Hazelnuts
Macadamia
Pecans
Pine nuts
Pistachios
Walnuts
NO PEANUTS! (They're not nuts—they're legumes.)

FRUIT (Yes, that's what they really are!)

Avocado (guacamole)
Olives (green and black)

OILS

On the Rosedale Diet, you will be eating lots of green salads. Use olive or avocado oil in your salad dressing. Steer clear of commercially prepared salad dressings that contain bad oils and are high in carbohydrate.

Almond oil
Avocado oil
Olive oil

FISH (highest in omega-3 fatty acids)

Halibut
Herring
Mackerel
Orange roughy
Sardines
Tuna

"A" List Protein Sources

EGGS (from algae or flax-fed chickens)

Omega-3 enriched eggs

FISH AND SEAFOOD (*especially good sources of omega-3 fatty acids)

Bass
Catfish
Cod
Crab
Flounder
Grouper
Haddock
Halibut*
Herring*
Lobster
Mackerel*
Mahimahi
Orange roughy*
Oysters (canned or fresh)
Perch
Pike
Pollack
Rainbow trout
Salmon* (canned or fresh)
Sardines* (canned in water, sardine oil, mustard, or olive oil)
Scallops
Shrimp (canned or fresh)
Snapper
Sole
Tilapia

Tuna* (canned or fresh)
Turbot

POULTRY (preferably free-range, organic)

Chicken breast, no skin
Ground chicken
Ground turkey
Chicken sausage
Turkey sausage

GAME

Cornish game hen
Buffalo
Ostrich
Pheasant
Rabbit
Venison

VEGGIE BURGERS (Look for low carb, high fiber burgers with no more than six carbs per burger.)

Chik Sticks Vegetable and Grain Protein Burgers
Morning Star Farms veggie sausage pattie
Natural Touch vegetable burgers

DAIRY

Goat cheese
No-fat cottage cheese
No-fat cream cheese
No-fat ricotta cheese
Feta cheese
Jarlsberg Lite Swiss cheese (great melted on a tortilla)
Parmesan cheese (one tablespoon per serving)

TOFU

Plain
Herb
Flavored (Italian, Oriental, Thai)

PROTEIN POWDER

Egg protein powder
Vegetable protein
Whey protein

"A" List Carbohydrate Sources

VEGETABLES

Asparagus
Artichoke hearts
Arugula
Bamboo shoots
Bell peppers (red, green, yellow, orange, hot)
Bok choy
Broccoli
Brussels sprouts
Cabbage
Cauliflower
Celery
Chard
Chives
Cilantro
Cucumbers
Endive
Eggplant
Fennel
Greens (collard, turnip, mustard, chard)

Hot peppers
Kale
Kohlrabi
Lettuce (all varieties except iceberg, which is low in nutrients)
Leeks
Mushrooms (portobello, shitake, oyster, button)
Okra
Onions
Parsley
Radicchio
Radishes
Rutabaga
Scallions
Seaweed (dulse, nori, hikiki, kombu)
Snow peas
Spinach
Sprouts (all varieties)
String beans
Turnip
Water chestnuts
Watercress
Zucchini

HIGH FIBER STARCHES

La Tortilla Factory tortilla
"Manna from Heaven" bread (¼ inch slice—contains 8 grams
   of protein, also counts as a protein)
Low carb, high fiber crackers (2–3 per day)

LEGUMES (eat in limited quantities)

Black soybeans
Hummus (made from chickpeas—as a condiment, not a meal)

COFFEE SUBSTITUTES

Roma
Teeccino
Cafix
Pero

TEA

Black tea
Green tea
Herbal tea

CONDIMENTS, SPICES, AND SEASONINGS

Basil
Bragg's Liquid Aminos (nonfermented soy sauce substitute)
Cardamom
Black pepper
Cayenne pepper
Capers
Cajun blended seasonings
Cinnamon
Crushed red pepper flakes
Cumin
Curry powder
Dill weed
Fennel
Garlic (fresh or powdered)
Ginger
Indian blended seasonings
Lemon
Lime
Mexican blended seasonings
Miso salt (if you are not on a salt restricted diet)
Mustard

Nutmeg
Onion (fresh or powdered)
Oregano
Paprika
Rosemary
Tamari
Tarragon
Thyme
Vanilla
Vinegar (balsamic, red wine, umeboshi [plum], and rice)
Worcestershire sauce

■ THE "B" LIST:

EAT THESE FOODS IN LIMITED QUANTITIES
AVOID THEM FOR THE FIRST THREE WEEKS ON THE DIET

"B" List Fat Sources

A splash of cream in your coffee or tea daily is allowed.
Butter for cooking
Canola oil
Coconut oil
Ghee (clarified butter for cooking)
High oleic safflower oil

"B" List Protein Sources

BEEF (no more than one serving twice a week)

Beef tenderloin
Cubed steak
Filet mignon

Flank steak
Ground round, extra lean
Ground sirloin, lean
Round steak
Roast beef (top round or rump)
Sirloin steak

LAMB (no more than one serving twice a week)

Chop
Leg
Roast

PORK

Lean, boiled ham
Loin chop
Pork tenderloin

DAIRY

Hard Cheese
Eat lite or low-saturated fat varieties of these in limited quantities (no more than one slice daily).

Cheddar
Colby
Havarti
Monterey Jack
Provolone
Swiss

Soft Cheese
Nonfat plain yogurt with one tablespoon of flaxseed to increase protein content (no more than two ½ cup servings per week).

One percent cottage cheese
Part skim milk ricotta cheese

"B" List Carbohydrates

VEGETABLES (no more than one serving [½ cup] per day and avoid for first two weeks)

Carrots
Parsnips
Peas

FRUIT (No more than one serving per day, ½ cup berries, ½ grapefruit, or one small piece of whole fruit. Use only fresh or frozen, not canned.)

Apples
Apricots
Blueberries
Cherries
Grapefruit
Kiwi
Nectarines
Peaches
Pears
Plums
Raspberries
Strawberries
Tomatoes

SEEDS (Preferably raw, unroasted and unsalted—I would much rather you eat nuts than seeds.)

Pumpkin
Poppy
Sesame

Sesame tahini (sesame paste)
Sunflower

LEGUMES

Adzuki
Navy
Lentil
Mung

LOW STARCH, HIGH PROTEIN PASTA

Keto spaghetti (low carb, high protein; just remember that the protein counts toward your daily total)

LOW CARB TOMATO SAUCE

Any brand with five or less grams of carbs.

BEVERAGES

1 cup of real coffee (for those who can't live without it)
4 ounces of red wine

SWEETENERS (in very limited quantities if you must)

Stevia
Sucralose

■ THE "C" LIST

TRY TO AVOID THEM ALTOGETHER

DAIRY

Milk (I'm not a fan of milk; see page 89.)
Frozen custard
Frozen yogurt
Fruit-flavored yogurt
Ice cream

ALL FULL-FAT HARD CHEESES (very high in saturated fat; if you happen to love a particular cheese, try to find a lite or variety lower in saturated fat)

Cheddar
Colby
Havarti
Monterey Jack
Provolone
Swiss

ALL CUTS OF MEAT NOT INCLUDED IN "A" PROTEIN OR "B" PROTEIN DELI MEATS (other than fresh cooked)

Chicken roll
Corned beef
Honey turkey
Hot dogs (all varieties including chicken and turkey)
Pastrami
Sandwich meats (bologna, salami, pimiento loaf, etc.)
Sausage (other than acceptable turkey or chicken sausage)
Turkey roll
Roast beef

OFF-LIMITS LEGUMES

Chickpeas (garbanzos) except for small amount of hummus
Lima beans
Peanuts
Peanut butter
Pinto beans

VEGETABLES

Corn and corn products (such as corn tortillas)
White potatoes (including powdered, mashed, fried, baked, etc.)
Pumpkin
Yams

ALL FRIED FOODS

Fried chicken
Fried fish
Chicken nuggets
French fries

BAD FATS

All commercially processed oils
Corn oil
Hydrogenated fats
Lard
Margarines with trans-fatty acids
Peanut oil
Safflower oil
Soybean oil
Sunflower oil
Squeezable butter or shortening

BAD CONDIMENTS

Barbecue sauce
Most commercially prepared salad dressings
Ketchup
Mayonnaise (unless made with good oils, such as olive oil, almond oil, avocado oil, or canola oil)

BEVERAGES

Fruit juice, all varieties
Soda pop, all varieties, diet or sweetened
Sports drinks
Sweetened teas

SUGAR AND ARTIFICIAL SWEETENERS (avoid foods containing the following ingredients)

Brown sugar
Corn syrup
Dextrose
Fructose
Honey
Maple sugar
Maple syrup
Nutrasweet
Saccharin
Sucrose
Sugar
Sweet'n Low
Turbinado

STARCHES

All bread (with the exception of "Manna from Heaven" bread or a comparable, very low-carb bread)

Couscous
Crackers (unless low carb and made with good fat)
Muffins
Packaged pancake mix
Packaged dry cereal (all brands)
Pasta
Rice
Quinoa
Waffles

FRUITS

Banana
Cantaloupe
Dried fruit (all varieties)
Grapes
Honeydew
Orange
Pineapple
Watermelon

SNACK FOODS

Chips (corn, potatoes, cheese, etc.)
Breakfast bars
Energy bars
Cakes
Candy
Cookies
Flavored Jell-O (sugar-free or regular)
Frozen fruit ice
Gelato
Ice cream
Popcorn
Pretzels

■ THE ROSEDALE DIET SAMPLE MEAL PLAN

Foods with accompanying recipes are designated by an asterisk. Recipes appear beginning on page 211 in the Resources section.

Please feel free to add a green salad with any or all of your meals.

■ ■ ■

DAY 1

Breakfast
Eggs "Benefit"*

Snack
Almonds

Lunch
Chicken Salad*

Snack
Avocado Spread on Celery Stalks*

Dinner
Dilled Salmon and Fresh Asparagus*
Salad of your choice

■ ■ ■

DAY 2

Breakfast
Nutola*

Snack
Celery with Almond Butter Stuffing*

Lunch
Salmon Salad*

Snack
Tamari Almonds*

Dinner
Baked Halibut with Green Beans*

■ ■ ■

DAY 3

Breakfast
Hard-Boiled Eggs and Swiss Chard*

Snack
Pumpkin Pecans*

Lunch
Tuna Salad*

Snack
Ginger Macnuts*

Dinner
Lobster Tails and Seaweed Salad*

■ ■ ■

DAY 4

Breakfast
Smoothie with Almonds*

Snack
Chai Nuts*

Lunch
Lobster Salad*

Snack
Almonds

Dinner
Grilled Tuna*

■ ■ ■

DAY 5

Breakfast
Avocado and Smoked Salmon Toasts*

Snack
Tamari Almonds*

Lunch
Maui Salad*

Snack
Black Soybean Dip* with crudités

Dinner
Garlic Shrimp*

■ ■ ■

DAY 6

Breakfast
Soft-Boiled Eggs Served Over "Manna from Heaven" Bread*

Snack
Walnuts

Lunch
Shrimp Wrap*

Snack
Cilantro Pesto Dip* with crudités

Dinner
Mung Dal Soup and Mesclun Salad*

■ ■ ■

DAY 7

Breakfast
Smoothie with Cashews*

Snack
Chai Nuts*

Lunch (begin to prepare in the morning after breakfast)
Gingery Chicken Soup*

Snack
Olive Tapenade* with crudités

Dinner
Tofu and Veggies in Lemon Tahini Sauce*

■ ■ ■

DAY 8

Breakfast
Eggs "Benefit"*

Snack
One slice of melted lite Jarlsberg cheese on a La Tortilla Factory
tortilla

Lunch
Spicy Chicken Salad*

Snack
Macadamia nuts

Dinner
Salmon Cakes with Asparagus*

■ ■ ■

DAY 9

Breakfast
Scrambled Tofu*

Snack
Walnuts

Lunch
Asparagus Soup and Deviled Eggs*

Snack
Avocado Spread* with crudités

Dinner
Chicken Tarragon*

■ ■ ■

DAY 10

Breakfast
Roasted Pepper Toasts*

Snack
Ginger Macnuts*

Lunch
Grilled salmon wrap with vegetables in a La Tortilla Factory tortilla

Snack
Basil Pesto Dip* with crudités

Dinner
Roasted Cornish Game Hens*

■ ■ ■

DAY 11

Breakfast
Smoothie with Hazelnuts*

Snack
Pumpkin Pecans*

Lunch
Romaine Salad à la Ron*

Snack
Spicy Cashews*

Dinner
Broiled Scallops*

■ ■ ■

DAY 12

Breakfast
Poached Eggs over Greens with Roasted Red Pepper Sauce*

Snack
Ginger Macnuts*

Lunch
Poached Salmon Salad*

Snack
Tamari Almonds*

Dinner
Baked Halibut in Pesto Sauce*

■ ■ ■

DAY 13

Breakfast
"Manna from Heaven" Bread with Pesto and Turkey Sausage*

Snack
Walnuts

Lunch
Cottage Cheese and Sautéed Kale*

Snack
Cilantro Pesto Dip* with crudités

Dinner
Curried Chicken*

■ ■ ■

DAY 14

Breakfast
Nutola*

Snack
Avocado Spread* with crudités

Lunch
Grilled salmon with vegetables in a La Tortilla Factory tortilla

Snack
Roasted Red Bell Pepper Dip* with crudités

Dinner
Grilled Mahimahi*

■ ■ ■

DAY 15

Breakfast
Eggs "Benefit"*

Snack
Macadamia nuts

Lunch
Sardines with mixed green salad

Snack
Chai Nuts*

Dinner
Trish's Tuna*

■ ■ ■

DAY 16

Breakfast
Toasted "Manna from Heaven" Bread with Avocado, Smoked Salmon,
Dill, and Poached Eggs*

Snack
Ginger Macnuts*

Lunch
Fish Chowder*

Snack
Walnuts

Dinner
Tofu Portobello Casserole*

■ ■ ■

DAY 17

Breakfast
Smoothie with Cashews*

Snack
Almonds

Lunch
Mesclun Mix Salad*

Snack
Walnuts

Dinner
Grilled Beef Fillets with Bell Peppers and Mashed Rutabagas*

■ ■ ■

DAY 18

Breakfast
Steak and Soft-Boiled Eggs*

Snack
Chai Nuts*

Lunch
Chicken Salad*

Snack
Tamari Almonds

Dinner
Turkey Burger, Mustard Greens, Feta, and Black Pepper*

▪ ▪ ▪

DAY 19

Breakfast
Poached Egg on "Manna from Heaven" Bread with Pesto*

Snack
Spicy Cashews*

Lunch
Grilled chicken with vegetables wrapped in a La Tortilla Factory tortilla

Snack
Pumpkin Pecans*

Dinner
Dijon Salmon served with Steamed Green Beans*

▪ ▪ ▪

DAY 20

Breakfast
Turkey Sausage with Poached Eggs*

Snack
Chai Nuts*

Lunch
Baby Romaine Salad*

Snack
Pumpkin Pecans*

Dinner
Grilled Chicken with Cilantro Pesto and Steamed Kale*

■ ■ ■

DAY 21

Breakfast
Berries and Yogurt*

Snack
Almonds

Lunch
Broccoli Soup*

Snack
Sardines and fresh crudités

Dinner
Halibut with Lime and Cilantro Served with Asparagus*

■ ■ ■

DAY 22

Breakfast
Eggs "Benefit"*

Snack
Tamari Almonds*

Lunch
Grilled Salmon and Steamed Chard*

Snack
Roasted Red Bell Pepper Dip* with crudités

Dinner
Pizza with Pesto Sauce*

■ ■ ■

DAY 23

Breakfast
Smoothie with Almonds*

Snack
Pistachios

Lunch
Country French Soup*

Snack
Celery with Almond Butter Stuffing*

Dinner
Black Cod*

■ ■ ■

DAY 24

Breakfast
Soft-Boiled Eggs and "Manna from Heaven" Bread with Sausage
Sauce*

Snack
Chai Nuts*

Lunch
Sea and Green Salad*

Snack
Your favorite mixed nuts

Dinner
Shepherd's Pie*

■ ■ ■

DAY 25

Breakfast
Smoked Salmon with Cream Cheese on "Manna from Heaven"
Bread*

Snack
Green and black olives

Lunch
Chicken Wrap*

Snack
Walnuts and blueberries

Dinner
Lasagna*

■ ■ ■

DAY 26

Breakfast
Berries and Yogurt*

Snack
Tamari Almonds*

Lunch
Lentil Soup*

Snack
Macadamia nuts

Dinner
Tilapia in Roasted Red Bell Pepper Sauce with Snow Peas*

■ ■ ■

DAY 27

Breakfast
Nutola* with cream

Snack
Your favorite dip and crudités

Lunch
Black Bean Wrap*

Snack
Pecans and walnuts

Dinner
Stuffed Peppers*

■ ■ ■

DAY 28

Breakfast
Smoothie with Hazelnuts*

Snack
Avocado Spread* with crudités

Lunch
Mesclun and Chicken Salad*

Snack
Macadamia nuts

Dinner
Country Buffalo Stew*

■ IN HIS OWN WORDS ■

P. L., AGE 52

"I had resigned myself to an early death. . . . Now I know each day is going to be a wonderful day."

I was diagnosed with type 2 diabetes in my forties, and had been following the traditional medical approach including medication and the American Diabetic Association diet, but nothing was working. I was just getting worse. I am a former dancer and used to be very active, but I was literally wasting away. When I first went to see Ron, I was down to 128 pounds and I'm six feet tall! I had lost much of the feeling in my legs from my knees on down. Things were getting very bad for me. My muscles had pretty much atrophied. I used to be able to do splits and bring my knees up to my head. It was just very distressing to not have any flexibility left.

I read about Ron and his different approach to treating diabetes in the local newspaper, so I figured, why not go see him? There was a lot of diabetes in my family. I'd pretty much given up hope because I'd seen my father die of the disease as had a couple of uncles and aunts. And I thought, well, you know, the natural progression, I guess, is to waste away, have your legs amputated, and then die. What I didn't realize is that they were not following any kind of diet, they were not strict with their medication or anything else. So they just wasted away. My outlook was pretty bleak until I went to see Ron.

Well, Ron actually guaranteed me that he could reverse my condition and I said, "Well, if you don't do it, do I have to pay you?" He said, "No!" Actually, Dr. Rosedale told me to go home and throw away my medication. He was so confident that he could reverse my diabetes. So I thought I'd try his program and see what happened. I went home and I emptied my cabinets, I emptied my pantry of all the processed, prepared food. Ron taught me how to read food labels. If a product had any kind of added sugar, I just threw it away. So I just threw everything out and went to the grocery store and bought only what was allowed on the program. I went into it with the attitude I'm going to do this 100 percent or not at all.

Within a short time, I stopped wasting away, and regained much of my strength. I've regained back all the feeling in my legs. Right now my weight is up to 160 pounds and I have about 8 percent body fat. I exercise at least six days a week, I just have so much energy! I never deviate from the diet—it makes me feel better so I stick to it. I can honestly say that I have not been sick with a cold or the flu since I started the regimen. It's just such a healthy way of eating.

People always comment on how healthy I look. They tell me that I just glow with good health. My whole attitude about life has changed; I wake up happy in the morning; I wake up smiling. Before, I had resigned myself to an early death. Now I know that every day is going to be a wonderful day.

chapter eight

A Guide to the Rosedale Diet Supplement Program

The cornerstone of the Rosedale Diet is diet, and as you get started on the program, you will see that food is very powerful medicine indeed. Although diet is the program's star, there are other tools that play important supporting roles. Exercise, of course, is very desirable, and so are targeted nutritional supplements, which we are going to focus on in this chapter. Let me make it clear up front that supplements are no replacement for a good diet. The Rosedale Diet can be effective without supplements, but supplements alone will not be particularly effective without the proper diet. That said, I believe that targeted nutritional supplements can dramatically enhance the effectiveness of the diet and will help you achieve your goals more rapidly. It may be hard to believe that something as simple as taking a few capsules a few times a day can make such a huge difference, but it can.

There are two separate supplement regimens: Rosedale Diet Supplement Plan is for people with mild metabolic dysfunction. This is for people who may be overweight, but who have not yet been diagnosed with a metabolic disease. Rosedale Diet Supplement Plan Plus is for people with more serious metabolic dysfunction. It includes many of the same supplements in the first program, but often at higher doses along with a few additional supplements. This is the program I use for patients who are extremely leptin and insulin resistant, diabetic, have poor blood lipid levels (such as high triglycerides), or have been diagnosed with heart and blood vessel disease. If you have a medical condition, please find a physician you can work with, and who can monitor you while you are on the Rosedale program. If you are taking medication for any of these conditions, you may be able to—and in some cases, absolutely must—dramatically cut back on your drugs after the good effects of the program kick in. Please consult your physician before making any changes in your drug regimen.

You can find the exact dosing information for each program starting on page 156.

▪ MULTIVITAMIN AND MINERAL SUPPLEMENT

Let's start with a multivitamin and mineral supplement. The chief function of vitamins and minerals is to serve as crucial constituents of enzymes or coenzymes, which facilitate chemical reactions throughout the body. Deficiencies of these key nutrients prevent enzymes from carrying out their functions. Take vitamin C, which is required by the enzymes involved in the production of collagen, the primary structural protein of our tissues. When vitamin C intake is inadequate, collagen synthesis is impaired. Blood vessels become fragile, wound healing is retarded, and skin and gums bruise and bleed easily. Vitamins and minerals may also have independent functions. Vitamin D, for example, directly helps regulate calcium metabolism. Whenever there is insufficient intake of vitamins and minerals, biological function falters.

You get lots of vitamins and minerals when you eat a healthy diet. However, government surveys suggest than fewer than a quarter of Americans meet even the bare minimum standards of a good diet (and believe me, the government's idea of a good diet is paltry indeed). We eschew nutrient-rich whole foods in favor of processed and prepared foods and eat out frequently, too often in fast-food restaurants. Furthermore, soil quality, storage conditions, and cooking methods may undermine the nutritional value of the food we eat, so there is no guarantee that you are getting all the nutrients you think you are getting. The rationale behind my recommendation for a good daily multivitamin and mineral supplement is to cover all your bases and make sure you get adequate levels of important nutrients.

I have three guidelines regarding multivitamin and mineral supplements. First, it's worth your while—and your money—to purchase a high-dose, high-quality product. Inexpensive one-a-day brands just won't do. Sure, they contain the recommended dietary allowances (RDAs) of the major vitamins and minerals, but, in my opinion, the RDAs are just too low. These minimum standards are designed "to meet the known nutritional needs of practically all healthy persons." But they ignore the mountains of research that show the therapeutic benefits of significantly higher doses, as we will discuss throughout this chapter. The brand we use at my clinic is normally a "six-a-day" supplement— more capsules, as you would suspect, are required to deliver higher, more reasonable levels of nutrients. Because you are also taking additional supplements, you only need to take four capsules of this multivitamin daily. How do you pick a multivitamin? Read the labels and find one that is close to the doses I recommend in this chapter.

See the Resources section for specific brand-name recommendations. (For the convenience of my patients, I have designed a line of supplements called Rosedale Metabolics that combine all my recommended supplements in several formulas. For more information on where to obtain them, see Resources. In this chapter, I give all recommendations for supplements in generic terms so you can purchase whichever products are most convenient and economical for you.)

Second, make sure your multi does not contain iron. Iron, unlike most other minerals, is not excreted but is stored in the body. High iron stores speed the production of free radicals and harmful oxidized LDL cholesterol, damage the arteries, and increase risk of heart attack. If you have iron-deficiency anemia, you can always add iron supplements, but this condition is relatively rare, except among women of childbearing age.

Third, when you have a choice between capsules and tablets, go for capsules. With tablets, you always run the risk that they are not going to dissolve; that they'll go right through you without being absorbed. This is not to say that all tablets are bad, but with gelatin capsules, you are guaranteed that they will break down and the contents will be released.

Most multivitamin and mineral supplements contain approximately twenty different nutrients. While all of them are beneficial, we will discuss in detail only those most important for the Rosedale Diet. Because various brands contain a wide range of doses, compare the amounts that your daily multivitamin and mineral provide of these key nutrients to my recommended doses, and, if necessary, beef it up with additional supplements. The usual dose for a good multivitamin and mineral supplement is two capsules, twice daily, with meals.

▪ ANTIOXIDANTS

As you know, the goal of the Rosedale Diet is to convert sugar metabolism to fat metabolism to turn you into a fat burner. But regardless of the fuel that is burned in the cells for energy, oxygen is usually consumed at the same time. A by-product of this reaction, which is called oxidation, is the production of free radicals: unstable molecules that attempt to stabilize themselves by stealing electrons from other molecules, destabilizing and damaging them in the process. Free radical destruction underlies virtually all degenerative diseases and the aging process itself.

You cannot stop the production of free radicals. They are an inevitable spin-off of energy generation. But you can slow down the rate at which they are produced by curbing your caloric intake or improving your metabolic efficiency via the Rosedale Diet, and you can dampen the damaging effects of free radicals by taking antioxidants. Antioxidants provide the electrons that free radicals are recklessly seeking and end their cycle of devastation. Some antioxidants, such as glutathione, are produced in the body. Others you get in your diet, especially when you eat lots of vegetables. However, to ensure optimal levels of these crucial compounds, it is important to take antioxidant supplements. Several antioxidants (such as C and E) are included in many multivitamins, but not at high enough doses to be effective. Others, that I consider to be extremely important for leptin sensitivity, such as lipoic acid, may not even be included. Let's focus on the most important antioxidants from the perspective of leptin resistance.

Vitamin C

Most people are familiar with vitamin C's immune boosting effects, popularized by the late Nobel laureate Linus Pauling, Ph.D. While vitamin C does play a vital role in immunity, protecting against cancer and viral and bacterial infections, it has multiple other functions as well. As I mentioned earlier, it is involved in collagen formation, so it speeds healing and slows the progression of arthritis and aging and it also helps detoxify heavy metals. Furthermore, vitamin C is the most active antioxidant in the aqueous, or water-based, portions of your body. Because of this, vitamin C's protective effects are widespread.

Vitamin C guards against free-radical damage to the arteries, thus warding off the first step in atherosclerosis and heart disease, which is an offshoot of the leptin resistance syndrome. In a 2001 study published in *The Lancet,* study participants with the lowest blood levels of vitamin C were two times more likely to die of heart disease as those with the highest vitamin C levels.

When blood sugar levels are high, as they often are in individuals with leptin resistance, intracellular levels of vitamin C are affected. In animals who produce vitamin C—and this includes all mammals with the exception of guinea pigs, one species of fruit-eating bats, and human beings and our fellow primates—this vitamin is actually derived from the glucose molecule. Similar to glucose, vitamin C requires insulin to gain entry into our cells. If the cells are resistant to insulin's signals, this vital nutrient cannot get in. Therefore, what may be an adequate dose of vitamin C for someone with normal glucose metabolism is inadequate for those with diabetes and insulin resistance. This partially explains the increased risk of infection among people with diabetes and those who eat a high-sugar diet—and why supplemental vitamin C boosts immune function.

Vitamin C also significantly slows glycation, the process by which glucose binds to proteins, interfering with their normal function. This process is accelerated by the elevations in blood glucose and body temperature typical of leptin resistance.

If you are following the Rosedale Diet Supplement Plan, I recommend that you take 250 mg. of vitamin C twice daily. If you are following the Rosedale Diet Supplement Plan Plus, I recommend that you take 500 mg. of vitamin C twice daily. If your multivitamin and mineral supplement contains less than what you should be taking, add enough vitamin C to achieve the recommended dose.

Vitamin E

Vitamin C's counterpart in the fat-based tissues is vitamin E: It is the body's premier lipid antioxidant. Fats are particularly prone to free-radical damage, and the resultant lipid peroxides are extremely harmful. Vitamin E prevents lipid oxidation. The high-fat diet that is part of Rosedale Diet necessitates the intake of high doses of this vitamin, for it prevents those fats from oxidizing.

One of vitamin E's primary purposes is to protect the unsaturated fats in the cellular membranes from oxidizing. It also prevents the oxidation of LDL cholesterol, which transforms this type of cholesterol into one of the major players in atherosclerosis. Combined with its other cardioprotective actions—it has a slight blood-thinning effect, discouraging the formation of blood clots, and helps relax the arteries—vitamin E is the guardian angel of the cardiovascular system.

Harvard researchers examined the effects of supplemental vitamin E in more than 87,000 female nurses and 46,000 male physicians and found that a minimum of 100 international units (IU) of vitamin E reduced risk of heart attack and death from heart disease by 37 percent in men and 40 percent in women, compared to those who took no vitamin E. And British researchers, in the double-blind placebo-controlled Cambridge Heart Antioxidant Study (CHAOS), concluded that taking 400 to 800 IU of vitamin E daily resulted in a 75 percent decreased risk of heart attack, compared to placebo.

Because vitamin E protects cellular membranes, it enhances the function of the receptors on the cells' surfaces that "hear" the signals of leptin, insulin, and other messengers. It has been shown to improve insulin sensitivity and glucose control and to lower fasting insulin concentrations. Vitamin E helps people with leptin and insulin resistance in another way as well: It dampens inflammation and lowers levels of highly sensitive C-reactive protein (CRP), which are often elevated in people with these conditions. Patients with diabetes are particularly likely to have elevations in this marker of inflammation and heart disease. Ishwarlal Jialal, M.D., and colleagues at the University of Texas Southwestern Medical Center in Dallas, treated patients with mild or severe type 2, insulin-resistant diabetes with 1,200 IU per day of vitamin E. They all had elevated CRP levels at the study's onset—twice the norm in those with severe diabetes and one-third higher than average in the mild diabetics. After three months of treatment, CRP levels had normalized in the patients with mild diabetes and fallen significantly in those with severe diabetes.

Vitamin E, even though it is a fat-soluble vitamin, is very safe—in fact, doses three times this high taken over extended periods have been shown to have no adverse effects. It is important that you take natural vitamin E, preferably with mixed tocopherols. On the Rosedale Diet Supplement Plan I recommend taking two 400 IU vitamin E capsules daily with food for a total of 800 IU. On the Rosedale Diet Supplement Plan Plus, I recommend taking three 400 IU vitamin E capsules daily for a total of 1200 IU. Very few multivitamin and minerals contain this level of vitamin E, so you will have to take extra E supplements.

Lipoic Acid

Lipoic acid, also called alpha lipoic acid, is an extremely versatile antioxidant. Unlike vitamin C, which scavenges free radicals from the watery areas of the body, and vitamin E, which is active in the lipids, lipoic acid is at home in both milieus. Furthermore, it works synergistically with both vitamin E and vitamin C, giving them a boost and sparing them for other functions.

Lipoic acid is also involved in energy production and particularly the metabolism of carbohydrates. All patients with diabetes, insulin resistance, and leptin resistance should take lipoic acid supplements. It helps lower blood sugar by improving insulin sensitivity, and equally important, it is highly effective in protecting against one of the most serious complications of elevated glucose: glycation. Lipoic acid is one of the most potent naturally occurring antiglycating agents. It is particularly helpful for diabetic neuropathy, nerve damage caused in part by glycation. At least fifteen clinical trials have examined the positive effects of high doses of lipoic acid in patients with diabetic neuropathy. In Germany, it is the treatment of choice for this condition. Among my own patients, I have seen severe neuropathy completely resolve with lipoic acid supplementation. Studies suggest that it is also protective of the eyes and may prevent diabetic retinopathy, cataracts, and other vision problems.

Lipoic acid has other, although unrelated, properties. One of these is heavy metal chelation. Its molecular structure and small size allow it to penetrate cell membranes and the blood-brain barrier, bind to heavy metals such as mercury, and remove them from the body. And because it protects against free radical damage to DNA, it has been used to treat victims of radiation exposure. When lipoic acid was given to children affected by the Chernobyl accident, it dramatically reduced markers of free radical damage. This supplement is extremely well tolerated and has very, very low toxicity.

B-Complex Vitamins

All multivitamin and mineral supplements contain folic acid, vitamin B12, vitamin B6, and other B-complex vitamins. These vitamins play a plethora of integral roles and are involved in immunity, reproduction, brain function, and, most important for our discussion, energy production and fat and carbohydrate metabolism.

One group of people—and this includes many with leptin resistance—needs to pay particular attention to their B-vitamin intake.

Those with elevations in homocysteine, a toxic by-product of protein metabolism, have a significantly increased risk of heart disease, Alzheimer's disease, cancer, and other serious conditions. Fortunately, an extremely effective means of lowering homocysteine is increasing your intake of folic acid, vitamin B12, and vitamin B6. The first two are key players in methylation, the process by which homocysteine is detoxified and cleared from the blood. Vitamin B6 plays an accessory role by converting homocysteine into cysteine, a harmless amino acid. If you do not have adequate amounts of these important vitamins at your disposal, methylation gets bogged down and blood levels of homocysteine rise. Methylation is also extremely important for genetic expression; inadequate amounts of folic acid is strongly linked to birth defects. Beef up these vitamins and homocysteine falls—it's as simple as that!

Biotin is another important B-vitamin that may not be present in your multivitamin and mineral supplement, at least not in therapeutic amounts. Biotin is involved in the metabolism of amino acids and essential fatty acids. It is particularly important for people with leptin and insulin resistance and diabetes, for it improves insulin sensitivity and helps lower blood sugar. Biotin stimulates the activity of an enzyme required for glucose utilization in the liver. When levels of this enzyme are low, glucose metabolism is impaired. Supplementing with high-dose biotin raises enzyme levels and has been shown to improve glucose control in both type 1 and type 2 diabetics.

In addition to what they are getting in their multivitamin, people following the Rosedale Diet Supplement Plan Plus program will need to take additional biotin.

■ MAGNESIUM

Magnesium is a key factor in hundreds of enzymatic reactions, helping to catalyze functions as diverse as cell replication, energy production, and protein synthesis. It helps regulate calcium metabolism and thus is involved in bone mineralization and the prevention of osteoporosis.

Magnesium also has a relaxing effect on the smooth muscle cells of the arteries, bronchioles, and skeletal muscles, and this gives it broad therapeutic powers. Supplemental magnesium dilates the arteries, lowering blood pressure and improving blood flow. It enlarges the airways, preventing and treating asthma attacks. It prevents spasms of the heart muscle and smoothes out irregular heartbeats. It even relaxes the muscles in the legs and arms, promoting a feeling of calmness and facilitating sleep.

It goes without saying then that magnesium deficiencies are closely linked with heart disease. But they are also associated with leptin and insulin resistance, as this mineral is very important for hormonal signaling. One of its most important functions is to repel calcium and keep it out of cells where in excess, it can do a lot of damage. In all but the minutest amounts calcium is a poison to all cellular life on earth and prevents proper hormonal communication.

In virtually all mineral supplements, the elemental mineral is attached to a binder that carries it across the intestinal lining so it can be absorbed by the body. Magnesium can be attached to several different binders, including aspartate, glycinate, and oratate. Read mineral labels carefully, because the doses indicated do not always reflect how much of the actual mineral the product contains. Labels should state the amount of elemental magnesium or the number of milligrams of magnesium as aspartate (or citrate, ascorbate, etc.). If it just says magnesium, it is referring to the total weight of the entire compound, so you have no idea how much magnesium you are actually getting, but it is definitely less than half of the total.

I recommend that you take 400 mg. of elemental magnesium daily. Your multivitamin and mineral will contain some magnesium, although it may be in a different form, which is fine. You will probably need to take additional magnesium supplements to reach 400 mg. daily. The only adverse side effect of magnesium is that it causes diarrhea in some people. If this is a problem for you, try 300 milligrams of magnesium or even less, if necessary.

P.S. The most absorbable form of magnesium is in green vegetables, from broccoli to lettuce to green peppers—so eat more of them!

■ ZINC

Zinc is another essential mineral that is a prerequisite for enzymatic reactions; it is involved in more than 200 such reactions in the body, ranging from protein metabolism and energy production to gene regulation and immune function. Zinc helps prevent birth defects, enhances sensory perception, and promotes mental alertness. Deficiencies are associated with immune dysfunction and impairments in vision, taste, and smell. Supplementing with zinc has been shown to prevent and slow the progression of macular degeneration, to enhance male fertility and prostate health, and to facilitate wound healing.

This mineral also plays a major role in the production of insulin in the pancreas and in the utilization of glucose by the cells. People with blood sugar and insulin abnormalities, which are quite common among those with leptin resistance, often have poor intestinal absorption of zinc, increased urine excretion, and low blood levels of this mineral.

Therefore, it is important for those with insulin resistance, diabetes, and other manifestations of leptin resistance to supplement with adequate amounts of zinc. There should be about 15 milligrams of zinc in your multivitamin. Those of you following the Rosedale Diet Supplement Plan Plus will need to supplement with additional zinc. Zinc should be balanced with copper, so select a supplement that contains 1 milligram of copper for every 15 milligrams of zinc.

■ CHROMIUM PICOLINATE

Chromium's importance in the regulation of blood sugar has been recognized since the 1950s, when U.S. Department of Agriculture researchers identified it as "glucose tolerance factor" because it so dramatically improved the activity of insulin and the uptake of glucose. Scores of clinical trials since then have elucidated chromium's sensitizing effects on the actions of insulin, and more than a dozen have demonstrated the benefits of chromium supplements for diabetes and insulin resistance. In one large double-blind placebo-controlled study conducted in China, 180 type 2 diabetics were divided into three groups and given either 200 or 1,000 micrograms supplements of chromium picolinate or a placebo per day, in divided doses. Then their average blood sugar levels were retested after four months, and the greatest benefits were observed in the patients taking the higher dose of chromium. Reductions were noted not only in blood sugar, but also in insulin, cholesterol, and glycated hemoglobin, a longer-term measure of blood sugar control and glycation.

Chromium has also been shown to facilitate weight loss and improve body composition by decreasing body fat and increasing muscle mass and may help curb appetite. I recommend 200 micrograms of chromium picolinate per day as part of the Rosedale Diet for everyone. Safety concerns about this well-absorbed form of chromium crop up every now and then, and if you have heard about them, I want to reassure you. A couple of test-tube studies have shown that when animal cells were exposed to extremely high levels of chromium picolinate—thousands of times the dose than a human would take—chromosomal damage occurred, as it could when exposed to high doses of any metal. I believe that these small studies do less to tarnish the reputation of this supplement than the reputations of the journalists who blew such insignificant results completely out of proportion. I am completely satisfied with chromium picolinate's safety and continue to recommend it as the preferred form of chromium.

Your multivitamin should contain 200 micrograms of chromium, which is what I recommend for the regular Rosedale Diet Supplement Plan. Those of you following the Rosedale Diet Supplement Plan Plus will need to take additional chromium supplements.

■ VANADYL SULFATE

Vanadium, a trace mineral named after the Nordic goddess of beauty and youth, is best known for its effects on glucose metabolism. Dozens of studies have shown that high doses of this mineral, usually in the form of vanadyl sulfate, improve fasting glucose and insulin sensitivity.

Debate continues as to exactly how vanadyl sulfate effects these improvements, but it appears to mimic the actions of insulin by directly stimulating receptors on the cells' surfaces (but apparently different receptors than those for insulin, thus reducing rather than worsening insulin resistance). Another interesting aspect of high-dose vanadyl sulfate is that its positive effects linger, sometimes for weeks after the supplement is discontinued.

Although the studies on high-dose vanadium are compelling, it may have some potential toxicity at higher doses—this is also an area of great debate among researchers. I don't prescribe vanadium for everyone, but primarily for my patients following the Rosedale Diet Supplement Plan Plus. I prescribe 15 milligrams of vanadyl sulfate daily, in divided doses with meals, which is a fairly low dose. I recommend a brand called Vanulin. (Diabetics will often be given temporary doses as high as 60 milligrams daily.) One possible side effect of this mineral is hypoglycemia, or low blood sugar, although I have rarely seen this in my patients at my suggested dose. This could be particularly problematic for people with diabetes who are taking medications to lower their blood sugars, which could be driven dangerously low. You should discuss this with your doctor if you are taking insulin or another diabetes drug. If you are affected by either of these side effects, cut back on your dose of vanadium.

■ GYMNEMA SYLVESTRE

Gymnema sylvestre is an herb that has been a standard of Ayurveda, the traditional medicine practice of India, since 600 B.C. It has three characteristics that make it an excellent supplement for anyone with impairments in blood sugar, insulin, or leptin regulation. First, the molecular structure of this herb resembles that of glucose, so it binds to receptors in the small intestine and decreases the absorption of glucose into the blood. Second, when applied directly to the tongue, it blocks the taste of sugar and may control appetite and sugar cravings. (This happens only when the herb directly contacts your taste buds, not when you take capsules or tablets of the herb.)

Third, *Gymnema sylvestre* improves blood sugar control by stimulating and possibly regenerating the beta cells in the pancreas. In a fascinating animal study, fasting glucose levels returned to normal and insulin production increased in insulin-dependent diabetic rats after treatment with *Gymnema sylvestre*. Incredibly, when the pancreases of these animals were examined on autopsy, the number of beta cells had doubled, compared to untreated animals. Several human studies have confirmed this herb's beneficial effects on the pancreas and glucose control. In one of these studies, type 1 diabetics taking an extract of this herb for six to eight months had average reductions in fasting blood sugar of 23 percent—and they were able to lower their insulin doses by one-quarter.

I only recommend *Gymnema sylvestre* for people following the Rosedale Diet Supplement Plan Plus program. Make sure you use a brand that is guaranteed to be standardized for 24 percent gymnemic acid (I would get the most gymnemic acids for the money, if from trusted companies), the herb's most active constituent. In recent years, quality manufacturers have begun selecting herbal extracts based on the concentration of their key ingredients. Standardized extracts have been analyzed and are guaranteed to contain a specific percentage of the compound believed to give the herb most of its therapeutic potential. Trying to select the best herbal products from all the tinctures, liquid extracts, capsules, and tablets derived from roots, leaves, flowers, or other sources that you find in health food stores can be overwhelming. This trend toward standardization is a godsend for consumers, for it ensures a degree of consistency.

My best advice is to purchase your products from a reputable company.

▪ COD LIVER OIL

With all the meat, dairy products, fried foods, and oils we eat, you might think that the last thing many of us would be low in is fat, but you would be wrong. The vast majority of Americans have deficiencies in one of nature's most essential fats: omega-3 fatty acids. If you never ate another bite of saturated or monounsaturated fat, your body would still be able to synthesize them from other fat and sugar. However, there are two types of fat that the body cannot manufacture, so they must be acquired from dietary or supplement sources. They are omega-3 and omega-6 essential fatty acids.

The reality is, most people eat too much omega-6s because they are quite abundant in the diet. If you eat nuts and seeds, vegetable oils, whole grains, and vegetables, you get plenty of omega-6 fatty acids. Omega-3s are another story, for they are abundant only in cold-water fish, marine mammals, and flaxseed oil. Since few people make a habit of eating any of these, deficiencies are rampant. This has created unhealthy imbalances in our cellular levels of fatty acids. Whereas an ideal ratio of omega-6 to omega-3 fats ratio is 1 to 1 or, at worst, 2 to 1, the average American's is in the neighborhood of 30 to 1!

Correcting this balance by taking supplemental cod liver oil will deliver a multitude of benefits. The EPA in fish oil subdues inflammation, smoothes out arrhythmias of the heart, protects the endothelial cells that line arteries, improves the elasticity of the arteries, prevents unwanted blood clots, enhances circulation, and importantly improves cellular hormone sensitivity. Fish oil's other primary fatty acid, DHA, nourishes the brain, lifts mood, and improves attention. The list of conditions that benefit from fish oil supplementation is exhaustive and includes diabetes, skin conditions, atherosclerosis, heart disease, rheumatoid arthritis and other inflammatory conditions, immune dysfunction, depression, bipolar disorder, and infertility—to mention just a few.

More germane to our discussion of leptin resistance are omega-3 fatty acids' effects on membrane and hormone receptor function. Taking omega-3 fatty acids will vastly improve membrane function and remarkably enhance insulin and leptin sensitivity. High doses of fish oil will also bring down triglycerides quickly and dramatically. In fact, when taken in conjunction with the Rosedale Diet, fish oil supplementation can cause triglycerides to plummet from the thousands to the low hundreds in just two or three weeks. Fish oil also stimulates the burning of fat, stoking the fire, so to speak, and facilitating the desired conversion from sugar burning to fat burning.

(For more information on the benefits of omega-3 fatty acids, see Chapter 5, "Why Good Fat Does a Body Good.")

Fish oil is a very important part of the Rosedale Diet. Although it is available in capsules, my favorite source is (filtered) liquid cod liver oil. I want you to take up to two tablespoons a day, depending on how much salmon and other omega-3-rich fish you eat. Before you turn up your nose at this suggestion, let me reassure you that gigantic strides have been made in the stabilization of fish oil in the last few years. Those of you who recall with disgust the rancid taste of the cod liver oil of your childhood will be pleasantly surprised by the mild taste of today's fish oil. I recommend Carlson's Norwegian Cod Liver Oil (lemon flavor), which is sold in many health food stores. Store it in the refrigerator after opening, and observe the product's expiration date, just as you would with a carton of milk. DO NOT USE IT AS A COOKING OIL.

▪ COENZYME Q10

Within nearly every cell are unique structures called mitochondria. They have their own unique DNA—distinct from cellular DNA—that is closely akin to a certain strain of bacteria. Strange as it may seem, scientists believe that at some time in the very, very distant past, ancient, bacterial relatives of modern mitochondria formed a symbiotic partnership with cells and became a part of them. This partnership was certainly a boon for the cell, for the mitochondria generate the bulk of the energy that fuels our cells.

Inside these little power plants, energy is produced in a complex process involving the burning of glucose and fat, the transfer of electrons, and the packaging of little chemical bundles of energy called ATP. One of the major players in what is known as the electron transfer chain is coenzyme Q10 (CoQ10). It makes sure that that energy transfer is efficient and does not leak into the cell and cause oxidative damage. Every cell that depends on mitochondrial energy production (the vast majority of cells on earth) also depends on CoQ10.

Supplemental CoQ10 enhances energy generation and also acts as a very potent antioxidant. Since muscles need lots of energy, it helps significantly in muscle contraction. It has been best studied as a treatment for various aspects of cardiovascular disease (remember that your heart is a muscle). It lowers blood pressure, reduces angina, or chest pain, and normalizes arrhythmia of the heart. CoQ10 is particularly useful as a treatment for congestive heart failure, which is characterized by a weakened, enlarged heart muscle with reduced pumping capacity. Patients with this condition are extremely fatigued, breathing is labored, and fluids collect in the lungs and extremities. According to conventional medicine, heart transplant is the only solution for patients with severe congestive heart failure. Yet CoQ10 is like a miracle drug for these patients. In a study published in the *American Journal of Cardiology,* taking CoQ10 dramatically reduced the average (quite high) death rate of patients with heart failure. Furthermore, it has taken many patients off heart transplant waiting lists. Alarmingly, the frequently prescribed statin drugs for lowering cholesterol deplete CoQ10 levels. If you are taking a statin cholesterol-lowering drug, it is imperative that you take supplemental CoQ10. These depletions are likely responsible for many of the adverse effects of the statin drugs, including muscle soreness and weakness and, in rare cases, complete muscle breakdown and death.

More recent coenzyme Q10 research has branched out into other areas. It has been shown to protect against cancer—and to promote tumor regression in some cases. High doses (1,200 milligrams daily) have dramatically slowed the progression of Parkinson's disease and other neurodegenerative disorders such as Huntington's disease. Migraine headaches, asthma, fibromyalgia, periodontal disease, cirrhosis of the liver: all of these conditions have responded to CoQ10 supplementation. Furthermore, because it helps maintain cellular energy production and protects the mitochondria, CoQ10 may actually retard aging.

I recommend that all my patients take 100 milligrams of coenzyme Q10 per day. This supplement is safe and well tolerated.

▪ L-CARNITINE

L-carnitine is also involved in energy production. It is required for the transport of fatty acids into the mitochondria, where they are burned for energy. If you do not have adequate carnitine, fat burning is impaired. Obviously, if you have leptin resistance and problems with burning fat, you want to make sure that plenty of carnitine is available to your cells.

The benefits of carnitine supplementation have been observed most frequently in the treatment of cardiovascular conditions because the heart, the busiest of muscles, loves to burn fat. This supplement has been demonstrated to reduce angina, improve heart function and exercise tolerance in patients with congestive heart failure, and speed up recovery from heart attacks. Carnitine's positive effects on fat metabolism also translate into lower triglyceride and cholesterol levels. In addition, there is some indication that it may improve exercise tolerance in healthy people, and many athletes take this supplement to improve physical performance. A form of carnitine called acetyl l-carnitine also protects mitochondrial membranes by protecting a vital component called cardiolipin and because of this, may show promise in extending life span.

Carnitine is better absorbed on an empty stomach, so I suggest taking it at least twenty minutes before breakfast and again at bedtime, two hours or so after eating. No toxicity or significant side effects have ever been reported with l-carnitine.

▪ L-ARGININE

The amino acid l-arginine is an important supplement for patients following the Rosedale Diet, especially those with any type of cardiovascular disease. Arginine is a precursor to nitric oxide (NO), the most potent vasodilator ever discovered. When NO is produced in the endothelial cells lining the arteries, it signals the arteries to relax and dilate. This increases blood flow, lowers blood pressure, and prevents arterial spasms. Arginine also protects the endothelial cells and prevents the formation of blood clots. Plaque-ridden arteries are unable to produce sufficient amounts of NO, which further accelerates atherosclerosis. Taking supplemental arginine helps restore endothelial function and improves several aspects of heart disease.

NO has tremendous therapeutic potential—and the drug companies have recognized this. Nitroglycerin, a common drug prescribed to patients with angina, works by increasing NO levels, which relaxes and enlarges the arteries and restores blood flow to the oxygen-starved heart muscle. Viagra, the blockbuster drug for erectile dysfunction, works by boosting NO levels that relax the arteries and improve penile blood flow. (Arginine supplements will help this condition as well, although not as dramatically as Viagra. If you are taking Viagra, talk to your doctor before using this supplement.)

In addition to its roles in circulation and cardiovascular disease, NO is also utilized by immune cells to dispatch bacteria and cancer cells. It serves as a neurotransmitter, or chemical messenger, in the brain. In addition, because arginine is easily glycated, it reduces the harmful effects of glycation in your body by acting as a sacrificial lamb, taking the hits that healthy cells would otherwise take and sparing them from glycation.

■ L-GLUTAMINE

L-glutamine is the most abundant amino acid in the blood. It is involved in the production of both glutathione, one of the body's most important antioxidants, and proteins. Because it promotes tissue regeneration, weight lifters often take this amino acid to hasten the repair of tissues that break down during intense exercise. One of glutamine's most important functions is to provide fuel for the mucosal and immune cells in the small intestine. Supplemental glutamine thus boosts immunity and improves gastrointestinal health by stimulating the growth of new mucosal cells, enhancing the integrity of the intestinal tract, and preventing leaky gut. This amino acid is particularly helpful for patients who have undergone surgery or trauma because it stimulates immune cell function and reduces the risk of infection by preventing bacterial translocations from the gut. Glutamine is useful for patients undergoing chemotherapy or radiation therapy, for it reduces the common gastrointestinal side effects of these therapies.

Glutamine is abundant in the brain and is one of the few things that can serve as a fuel for the brain in the absence of glucose. It helps stabilize blood sugars and is particularly useful in fending off hypoglycemia, or low blood sugar. Moreover, glutamine decreases sugar and alcohol cravings, likely due to its stabilizing effects on blood sugar.

I recommend that you take 2,000 milligrams of glutamine before you go to bed at night. Your immune system is most active when you sleep, so this is a good time to fuel up the immune cells in the intestines and to boost glutathione levels. If you are experiencing sugar or alcohol cravings, take up to 500 milligrams of glutamine two or three times during the day as needed (up to 2,000 milligrams) as long as you lower your nighttime dosage accordingly. The most effective means of curbing cravings is to use a powdered form of glutamine mixed in water (it tastes fine), or open a capsule and let it dissolve on your tongue. Amino acids are best taken on an empty stomach, twenty minutes before meals or two hours after meals. Glutamine may be taken with a little fat, but for maximum absorption, avoid taking it with protein.

▪ PHOSPHATIDYLSERINE

Phosphatidylserine is a phospholipid, a fat-phosphorus compound that makes up the bulk of our cellular membranes. Phosphatidylserine is particularly abundant in the brain where it is incorporated into the cell membranes of neurons and thus plays a major role in nerve cell function.

Supplemental phosphatidylserine easily crosses the blood-brain barrier, the cellular and chemical "bouncers" that control what goes into and out of the brain. This is important, because some nutritional supplements claimed to nourish the brain are not even allowed in.

Approximately 3,000 studies have examined the workings of this phospholipid, and scores of clinical trials demonstrate the beneficial effects of supplemental phosphatidylserine on age-related declines in memory and learning. In one remarkable twelve-week study of fifty- to seventy-year-olds with minor memory impairment, it was shown to dramatically improve ability to memorize text, recall phone numbers, remember names and faces, locate misplaced objects, and concentrate. In fact, the study subjects taking this supplement performed as well as people twelve years their junior.

Phosphatidylserine is incorporated into cell membranes outside the brain as well, and thus it improves sensitivity to leptin, insulin, and other hormones. In addition, it reduces the conversion of muscle tissue into blood sugar.

Although this supplement would be beneficial for everyone, it's imperative for people following the "Plus" Plan.

■ PREGNENOLONE

Pregnenolone is a steroidal hormonal produced in the adrenal glands. It is sometimes referred to as the "mother hormone," because it is a precursor to DHEA, progesterone, estrogen, testosterone, and cortisol. Because it can allow for the manufacture of cortisol, it can help with "adrenal fatigue" often seen in diabetes and other metabolic "high stress" disorders. High leptin levels as seen in leptin resistance leads to chronic overstimulation of the sympathetic nervous system, predisposing to adrenal fatigue and "burnout," with abnormally low cortisol. Yet pregnenolone has independent functions of its own. Produced in the brain and the cells of the spinal cord as well as the adrenal glands, it activates both receptors that stimulate the brain and receptors that calm it. Therefore, pregnenolone has a beneficial, stabilizing effect on brain function.

Animal studies suggest that supplemental pregnenolone is a highly effective memory booster. Small human studies also show encouraging benefits in improving concentration, reducing mental fatigue while performing stressful tasks, and elevating mood.

Pregnenolone production, like that of all steroidal hormones, declines with age, and I particularly recommend it for people over age fifty. This supplement is not part of the regular supplement plan, but is recommended for those following the "Plus" Plan.

▪ GETTING STARTED

Many of the nutrients on this list may be taken in combination form. As I mentioned above, vitamins C and E, the B-complex vitamins, magnesium, zinc, and chromium will all be found in multivitamin and mineral supplements—albeit not necessarily in the doses I recommend.

Some of the other supplements—*Gymnema sylvestre,* vanadyl sulfate, chromium picolinate, and lipoic acid—are often combined, along with other glucose-lowering and insulin-sensitizing nutrients, in products formulated for diabetics. So if you shop around, you should be able to find combination products that contain several of these different supplements. I have designed my own combination formulas. For more information, see the "Rosedale Resources" section.

Another concern you may have when looking at this list is, "How long do I have to take all these supplements?" I want you to be extremely vigilant during the first three months of the program. After that, provided that your leptin levels have normalized and other metabolic problems have resolved, you can taper off some of the "accessory nutrients." For example, unless a patient has diabetes, *Gymnema sylvestre* and vanadyl sulfate may be discontinued and the dose of chromium lowered after three months. As sugar cravings subside, l-glutamine can be stopped. Biotin can be lowered or discontinued also.

I believe that everyone benefits from a daily multivitamin and mineral supplement, and I recommend that such a supplement be taken indefinitely. Other nutrients on the list, including l-carnitine and coenzyme Q10, have exceptional benefits and, if you can afford them, I would suggest staying on them as well. In fact, there is certainly no harm in taking the entire list for the rest of your life (except perhaps for vanadyl), and each and every one of them does offer significant benefits. But no, it isn't imperative that you take all of them indefinitely.

■ THE ROSEDALE DIET SUPPLEMENT PLAN

UPON WAKING, BEFORE BREAKFAST

SUPPLEMENT	DOSAGE
L-Arginine (Take on an empty stomach)	1,000 mg.
L-Carnitine (Take on an empty stomach)	1,000 mg.

WITH BREAKFAST

SUPPLEMENT	DOSAGE
Chromium Picolinate	200 mcg.
Coenzyme Q10	100 mg.
Cod Liver Oil (liquid only)	1 Tbs.
Lipoic Acid	200 mg.
Magnesium Potassium Aspartate	500 mg.
100 mg. Magnesium	
99 mg. Potassium	
301 mg. Aspartate	
Multivitamin (no iron)	(2) capsules
Vitamin C	250 mg.
Vitamin E	800 IU

WITH DINNER

SUPPLEMENT	DOSAGE
Lipoic Acid	200 mg.
Magnesium Potassium Aspartate	1,000 mg.
Multivitamin (no iron)	(2) capsules
Vitamin C	250 mg.

AT BEDTIME

SUPPLEMENT	DOSAGE
L-Arginine	1,500 mg.
L-Glutamine Powder	½ tsp.
L-Carnitine	500 mg.

For optimal absorption, make sure your stomach is empty—take it twenty minutes before eating or at least two hours after eating. If it causes stomach upset, which it does in some people, try it with a little fat-containing food, but avoid eating protein at the same time you take arginine. If you use Viagra or nitroglycerin, talk to your doctor before taking arginine. Also talk to your doctor if you are pregnant or have an autoimmune disease, migraine headaches, AIDS, cirrhosis, depression, or breast cancer, for this supplement may not be appropriate for people with these conditions.

■ THE ROSEDALE DIET SUPPLEMENT PLAN PLUS

UPON WAKING, BEFORE BREAKFAST

SUPPLEMENT	DOSAGE
L-Arginine (Take on an empty stomach)	2,000 mg.
Acetyl-L-Carnitine (Take on an empty stomach)	1,000 mg.

WITH BREAKFAST

SUPPLEMENT	DOSAGE
Biotin	7.5 mg.
Chromium Picolinate	400 mcg.
Coenzyme Q10	100 mg.

Cod Liver Oil (liquid only)	1 Tbs.* For first three weeks, take 2 Tbs.
Gymnema Sylvestre Extract	500 mg.
Lipoic Acid	300 mg.
Magnesium Potassium Aspartate	1,000 mg.
100 mg. Magnesium	
99 mg. Potassium	
301 mg. Aspartate	
Multivitamin (no iron)	(2) capsules
Phosphatidylserine	200 mg.
Pregnenolone	50 mg.
Vanadyl Sulfate	20 mg.*
Vitamin C	500 mg.
Vitamin E	1,200 IU
Potassium Aspartate	200 mg. (for first three weeks only)

*Take for first three months, stop if blood sugar drops too low.

WITH DINNER

SUPPLEMENT	DOSAGE
Biotin	7.5 mg.
Chromium Picolinate	400 mg.
Gymnema Sylvestre Extract	500 mg.
Lipoic Acid	300 mg.
Magnesium Potassium Aspartate	1,000 mg.
Multivitamin (no iron)	(2) capsules
Potassium Aspartate	200 mg. for first three weeks only
Vitamin C	500 mg.
Phosphatidylserine	200 mg.

AT BEDTIME

SUPPLEMENT	DOSAGE
L-Arginine	2,000 mg.
L-Glutamine Powder	½ tsp.
Acetyl-L-Carnitine	500 mg.
Magnesium Potassium Aspartate	500 mg.

A note on arginine: For optimal absorption, make sure your stomach is empty. Take it twenty minutes before eating or at least two hours after eating. If it causes stomach upset, which it does in some people, try it with a little fat-containing food, but avoid eating protein at the same time you take arginine. If you use Viagra or nitroglycerin, talk to your doctor before taking arginine. Also talk to your doctor if you are pregnant or have an autoimmune disease, migraine headaches, AIDS, cirrhosis, depression, or breast cancer, for this supplement may not be appropriate for people with these conditions.

■ IN HER OWN WORDS ■

S. K., AGE 63

"I lost 25 pounds . . . and I actually gained back some bone and muscle."

I had a hysterectomy at age forty, it really changed my body. The pounds started to creep up on me. When I was in my fifties, I had a bone scan that showed signs of osteoporosis, so my doctor put me on estrogen replacement therapy to try to prevent more bone loss. I had also developed high blood pressure, and was taking a diuretic that helped to bring it down. I was trying to lose weight by following a strict low fat diet. I would snack on pretzels because they had 0 grams of fat, and eat lots of carbs as long as they had no fat, but I kept gaining weight. I went to see Ron because I wanted to try a different approach, and I wasn't feeling very well. I felt tired all the time, and about two hours after I would eat breakfast, I would get light-headed and dizzy. There were days that I felt so bad that I was just miserable! At the initial visit, Ron did some tests, and found that I had high blood sugar and elevated leptin levels. Ron put me on the opposite diet to one that I was eating—very few carbs (other than vegetables) and lots of good fat—and put me on a supplement program. After I started the diet, Ron took me off all my medication, and I began to feel better pretty quickly. The first thing that I noticed was that I had a lot more energy. I lost about twenty-five pounds—losing the weight was easy—and I actually gained back some bone and muscle, which made me very happy. My primary exercise is walking, and I'm now able to walk much farther than I did before. I feel a lot stronger, a lot lighter and a lot healthier.

chapter nine

Rosedale Diet Exercise Strategies

I know what many of you are thinking. Like in so many other diet books, this is the part of the book (buried at the very end) where you expect me to finally level with you and confess that unless you're willing to commit hours a day to pumping iron, or running marathons, or jumping rope until you're ready to drop, my program isn't going to work and you're always going to be fat. So, those of you who expect to hear the worst, you're in for a pleasant surprise. This chapter is short and to the point, which is just what I think exercise should be.

Based on the experience of thousands of patients, I can say with utmost certainty that if you follow the Rosedale Diet, you will achieve excellent results even if you never pick up a weight or dust off your treadmill. Once you regain your leptin sensitivity, your body will start burning off excess fat, and you will maintain muscle and lean mass. You will look trim and sleek because you are finally eating the way you should be eating and you will no longer be weighed down by all that fat.

The major benefit of lots of exercise is that it covers up many dietary mistakes. If you are eating a diet that converts much of the food that you eat (either starch or excess protein) into sugar, it is far better to burn it off by exercising than to leave it around to raise leptin and insulin levels. In this way, you can lessen damage done by poor diet, but you cannot negate it. It is wiser to avoid eating the wrong food in the first place. The Rosedale Diet makes exercise less necessary; however, adding some mild exercise while following the Rosedale Diet can take you to another level that can't be achieved on other programs.

Many patients have told me that they have exercised until they were "blue in the face" but have barely lost any weight, and continue to feel flabby. The reason for this is simple. Exercise without the proper metabolic instructions to burn fat and build muscle leads to very disappointing results. By following the Rosedale Diet you will correct leptin and insulin signaling and therefore, the metabolic signals necessary to achieve optimal results from exercise.

Diet is the linchpin of my program; exercise is of lesser importance. I'm not saying exercise is bad. It's great if you like to do it, and if you do it sensibly and in moderation so that you don't injure or overstress your body. Exercise usually lowers blood sugar and has been proven to lower leptin levels and increase insulin sensitivity. It improves circulation, which helps transport nutrients to your cells so that they can get adequate nourishment. And it makes you feel good. These are good reasons to exercise and I certainly recommend it. It contributes to optimal results on my program and can make the regimen easier. Actually, I consider exercise to be a very good "supplement" to my program. I hope that people do it, but the program will usually still work if they don't as long as they are extra diligent about following the rest of the program's guidelines.

The other reason that I don't overemphasize exercise is that I don't want people to become overly reliant on using exercise as the primary tool to maintain weight loss, since exercise without proper diet is woefully inadequate. Also, I have noticed that very few patients actually make lasting improvements in their exercise habits.

So, my goal is to make exercise easy for you. I recommend around fifteen to twenty minutes of exercise daily—not necessarily more—of doing something that you like to do. Ideally, you should exercise after your evening meal so that you can burn up every drop of excess sugar from dinner before you go to sleep. No matter how well you eat, you'll

EXERCISE AS A "MORNING-AFTER PILL"

If you *occasionally* slip up and eat a meal that contains too many sugary or starchy carbs, you can compensate by doing your fifteen-minute exercise regimen immediately after eating. This will help burn up the sugar before it raises your leptin and insulin levels, and is being stored as fat on your tummy, thighs, or rear end. Remember, though, that working your body too hard can be even more damaging than working it too little, particularly for people who are insulin resistant or are diabetic. A high-intensity workout can rev up production of stress hormones and cause blood glucose levels to rise as a result of tearing down excess muscle mass to burn as fuel. This is particularly damaging for someone who is insulin resistant, and is more likely to burn sugar and store fat.

still have some sugar that you need to burn off. Even broccoli contains some sugar! So try to burn off any excess long before your head hits the pillow. (Remember, your last meal should be about three hours before bedtime.) That way, it will be easier for your body to stay in fat burning mode for the duration of the night, while you sleep. If you can't bear to exercise in the evening, you can do your fifteen minutes during the day. The one thing that you absolutely should NOT do at night is eat a big meal and then lie down on the couch to sleep it off. That will keep you in sugar burning mode–fat storage mode and you will not lose as much body fat.

My only requirement is that you choose an exercise or regimen that involves some resistance training, and that engages your big muscle groups (legs and stomach in particular). This would automatically also be somewhat aerobic, which works your heart muscle and cardiovascular system. For example, a brisk walk in a hilly area is a great way to exercise major muscle groups and get a good aerobic workout. If you prefer, you can walk on a treadmill set on an uphill setting or use a stationary bicycle set on higher resistance (either at home or at the gym) for fifteen minutes, or you can spend fifteen minutes in front of the TV doing sit-ups, push-ups, and bicep curls with a set of light weights. You can change your fifteen-minute workout every day, if you like. My point is, there are no hard and fast rules, but you should do something at a moderately vigorous level for fifteen minutes each day. How do you know if you're working at the right level? You should be breathing somewhat faster, but you should still feel comfortable and not overtaxed. Breaking a light sweat is good; feeling overcome by heat or being drenched in sweat is bad. If your heart is pounding and you feel exhausted or dizzy, you are working with too much intensity. (If you feel chest pains, nausea, or sick when you work out, call your doctor immediately.)

■ EXERCISE AS A TOOL TO RELAX

Exercise need not be stressful. The right exercise can promote relaxation. For example, I have directed many of my patients to yoga classes, where they do gentle stretching exercises along with learning relaxation techniques. For those of you unfamiliar with yoga, it's a discipline that originated in India many thousands of years ago. It incorporates yoga postures (asanas) that exercise and stimulate every part of the body, especially stretching and toning muscles and joints. Yoga breathing exercises are known as pranayanas. They help relax and revitalize the body. There are several different types of yoga, including so-called power yoga that gives an intense workout. I recommend that you stick to the more traditional yoga that emphasizes mild stretching, relaxation, and deep breathing as opposed to the more aggressive versions.

In addition to making you feel good, yoga offers concrete health benefits. Recent studies confirm that yoga positions can lower high blood pressure, reduce your heart rate and improve arthritis, among other ailments.

The point to remember about exercise is that you don't have to spend hours at the gym forcing yourself to undergo strenuous exercise to achieve tremendous results. A nice walk after dinner over hills and dales, remembering to stop and smell the roses, is just fine while on the Rosedale Diet.

chapter ten

The Leptin Test and Other Medical Tests That Can Save Your Life

How will you know if the Rosedale Diet is working for you? The way you look and feel and the amount of weight you lose are the most visible signs that you are increasing your leptin sensitivity. I also recommend, however, that you get the laboratory tests discussed in this chapter prior to starting the Rosedale Diet and do the appropriate follow-ups after three months, six months, and one year, or as indicated. Just as your doctor periodically checks your cholesterol, I much prefer to follow other laboratory tests that I feel are far more indicative of your overall health. These will provide concrete, irrefutable proof of the program's beneficial effects on your overall health.

Of the sixteen medical tests described below, at least seven can be included as part of the routine CBC, or complete blood chemistry, that should be done at your annual physical. (An asterisk designates the tests that can be included as part of this routine workup.) Most of these tests require a blood sample drawn from a vein on the inside of the elbow or the back of the hand. Don't worry, the lab can use the same blood sample for several tests, which means that your doctor is not going to have to take more than a few blood samples. Because some tests require a fasting blood sample, you will be instructed by your doctor to avoid eating or drinking anything besides water for at least eight hours prior to having your blood drawn. Several of the tests described below are outside the range of the usual blood tests and should be sent to one of a handful of specialized labs for analysis. (See the "Rosedale Resources" section for lab recommendations.)

The tests are listed below in what I consider to be their order of importance.

Leptin
Insulin
HbgA1c
Glucose*
Thyroid function
Basal temperature
IGF-1
Norepinephrine
C-reactive protein
Triglycerides*
Homocysteine
BUN*
Creatinine*
Uric acid*
Liver enzymes*
Cholesterol*

■ LEPTIN

The most reliable test for monitoring leptin levels is the radioimmunoassay (RIA), which utilizes an antibody that responds to leptin in a fasting blood sample. This test will tell you whether or not you have leptin resistance. **If your level is in a healthy range—the optimal fasting leptin level is between 4 and 6 ng/dL and up to 9 ng/dL is acceptable—your cells are sensitive to leptin's signals.** You are a fat burner as nature intended you to be, and it is unlikely that you will have a weight problem. (If you lower your leptin levels to optimal levels, as you most certainly will on the Rosedale Diet, it is highly unlikely that you will continue to have a weight problem even if you started out with one.) Of course, we don't want leptin levels to go too low. Anything below −4 ng/dL is a sign of either malnutrition, usually accompanied by very low body fat, or a genetic inability to produce leptin that results in obesity. (If a woman's leptin level falls below 3, generally caused by very low stores of body fat due to inadequate food intake or intensive exercise, she will stop menstruating.)

If your fasting leptin level is 10 ng/dL or higher, you will most certainly benefit from the leptin-sensitizing program outlined in this book. Most obese people have extremely elevated leptin levels: 20, 30, even 40 ng/dL! Yet within only two to three weeks on the Rosedale Diet, almost everyone experiences a dramatic decline in leptin levels. At the same time, they eat less because they do not feel hungry as often as they used to. They no longer experience food cravings and have little difficulty following the diet. If your leptin level doesn't fall as quickly as it should (younger people often have quicker results than older people), you need to be especially careful about following the diet and perhaps add extra nutritional supplements. But if you follow the program, I promise that your leptin sensitivity will improve and your fasting leptin level will fall.

Leptin: 4 to 6 ng/dL optimal; up to 9 ng/dL acceptable; 10+ ng/dL high.

■ INSULIN

The most important test after leptin is fasting insulin, for this hormone is also involved in how your body utilizes energy. Insulin is best known for its effect on blood sugar. Secreted by specialized cells in the pancreas, called islet cells, in response to increases in blood glucose, insulin binds to receptors on the surfaces of cells throughout the body and signals them to allow glucose to enter.

Insulin regulates the energy needs of nearly every cell in your body. In addition to clearing glucose out of the blood, it determines whether that glucose will be used for immediate energy needs, whether it will be converted into glycogen for use over the next few hours, or whether it will be converted into fat for future needs. This explains why elevated insulin and leptin resistance go hand in hand in promoting weight gain. It is also involved in the synthesis of protein.

It is easy to overlook the manifold actions of insulin because its blood sugar–influencing properties are all you hear about from your doctor and the media. But let's look at it from an evolutionary perspective. For most of human history, the challenge was uncertain access to a food supply of any kind. Storing nutrients for times of food deprivation was essential to survival, and this is exactly what insulin does. Thus, insulin lowers blood sugar secondary to its major role in trying to store excess sugar mostly as fat.

Unfortunately, the fine-tuned processes that kept us alive during times of scarcity are undermined by our present diet that keeps blood levels of insulin constantly elevated.

One of the earliest effects of excess insulin is weight gain, as it stimulates the storage of fat and the burning of sugar. It lowers cellular levels of magnesium, a mineral that relaxes the arteries and improves blood flow. Insulin also increases accumulations of sodium, causing fluid retention, resulting in high blood pressure. Elevated insulin also increases inflammatory compounds in the blood that damage the arteries and promote the formation of blood clots that may cause a heart attack. It stimulates spasms in the arteries and arrhythmia in the heart. Furthermore, it causes abnormalities in blood fats, including reductions in protective HDL cholesterol and elevations in triglycerides and small, dense LDL cholesterol. All this translates into a significant increase in risk of heart disease.

There's more. Excess insulin upsets hormonal balance and increases the risk of polycystic ovary disease. It is even strongly linked to cancer because of its role in cell proliferation. Finally, high levels of insulin interfere with the normal activity of leptin with very few exceptions; if you are insulin resistant, you are also leptin resistant.

The best way to determine if you are insulin resistant is to have a fasting insulin test to measure total and/or free fasting insulin in serum. Free insulin is the active form of insulin, not bound to antibodies or other proteins, and levels will be slightly lower than total insulin. Ideal levels are less than 10 IU/mL. Anything above this means you are insulin resistant—and the higher your level, the more severe the condition. If your insulin is creeping toward 10 IU/mL, you have a window of opportunity to take steps to improve your insulin sensitivity. If your level is above 10 UU/mL, it is imperative that you do what it takes to get insulin resistance under control.

Because insulin resistance and leptin resistance are so closely intertwined, insulin levels respond beautifully to the Rosedale Diet. As you adopt the diet, supplement, and exercise recommendations outlined in this book, your cells become more sensitive to insulin and your insulin level will drop. At the same time you will be losing weight, reducing your risk of diabetes, heart disease, cancer, and other ills, and setting the stage for a long and healthy life.

Fasting Insulin: 10 IU/mL and below optimal; over 10 IU/mL high.

■ HBGA1C (GLYCATED HEMOGLOBIN)

Glucose, as we discussed in earlier chapters, interacts with proteins in a process called glycation, or glycosylation. When that protein is hemoglobin, the iron-carrying pigment that gives red blood cells their color, the end result is glycated hemoglobin (HbgA1c). (We could measure glycation in other blood proteins such as albumin, but this is the most economical and universally accepted test.)

The HbgA1c test, which measures the percentage of hemoglobin that is glycosylated, is used by most doctors to estimate average blood sugar levels over the preceding 120 days (the average life span of a red blood cell). If your HbgA1c is 5.5 percent, this means your average fasting blood sugar for the past three months was approximately 100 mg/dL. An HbgA1c of 8 percent translates into average blood sugars of approximately 200 mg/dL, and 11 percent into approximately 300 mg/dL.

As opposed to measuring average blood sugars, this test really reveals the rate of glycation, and glycation can be modified especially by taking certain supplements. I have seen patients with similar blood sugars, yet one may have a HbgA1c of 6 percent while the other's is 7 percent. This is very important, for if diabetic patients can keep their glycation levels low they are that much less likely to be afflicted with complications of the arteries, nerves, eyes, and kidneys—regardless of their glucose control. The nondiabetic HbgA1c range is from 4.5 to 6 percent, and the lower the level, the better.

There are several things you can do to curb glycation and lower HbgA1c. First, lower you blood sugar by changing your diet and improving your leptin and insulin sensitivity. Second, take targeted nutritional supplements, as we discussed in Chapter 8. Finally, reset your thermostat and lower your basal body temperature (by lowering leptin), for higher temperatures accelerate glycation. All of these very important changes can be made by implementing the Rosedale Diet.

HbgA1c: 5.4 or less percent optimal; 5.6–5.8 percent acceptable; 5.9 to 6.9 percent high; 7.0 or higher at risk of diabetic complications.

■ GLUCOSE

A fasting glucose test measures the amount of glucose, or sugar, in your blood. Most of the carbohydrates you eat are broken down into glucose and released into the bloodstream. Some of that glucose is burned for energy. Excesses are either stored in the liver and muscles in the form of glycogen for short-term energy needs or converted into fat for long-term storage.

Glucose testing is commonly used to screen for diabetes and to monitor blood sugars in people who have diabetes. Most physicians consider normal levels to be up to 110 mg/dL. A diagnosis of diabetes is made when fasting glucose is higher than 125 mg/dL. Levels between 110 and 125 mg/dL are indicative of impaired glucose tolerance, often called prediabetes. I think we need to redefine normal; normal is not necessarily healthy. If your glucose level is in the 70s or low to mid 80s, fine, but if it is in the 90s or above, you need to take steps to address the underlying hormonal imbalances that are driving your blood sugar up.

The Rosedale Diet has a tremendous effect on glucose levels. By avoiding carbohydrates and excessive proteins and adding more healthy fats to your diet, you can avoid dramatic spikes in glucose (not to mention insulin and leptin)—and the stresses that these unnatural spikes place on your energy-regulating systems.

Glucose: 70 to 85 mg/dL optimal; 85 to 110 mg/dL high; 110 to 126 mg/dL very high; 126+ mg/dL indicative of diabetes

■ THYROID FUNCTION TESTS (FREE T3, TSH)

Any discussion of metabolism must include the thyroid, a small gland located in the neck, straddling the windpipe. The thyroid produces two hormones, thyroxine (T4), and triiodothyronine (T3). Although the gland secretes much more T4 than T3, T3 is the more active of the two—T4 is converted to T3 in tissues throughout the body, mostly in the liver. Thyroid hormone affects almost every cell in the body. It stimulates enzymes involved in the oxidation, or burning, of glucose in the cells and controls the body's metabolic rate and production of body heat.

When the thyroid produces excessive amounts of hormones, the body runs hot, like a car idling too high. Body temperature is elevated, basal metabolism revs up, and fuel is rapidly burned up. It wears down the engine and wastes energy. Enormous appetite, insomnia, palpitations (strong or irregular heartbeat), trembling of the hands, irritability—these are all symptoms of excessive thyroid hormone levels, or hyperthyroidism.

An underactive thyroid, or hypothyroidism, causes an excessive slowdown in metabolism accompanied by too low temperature, fatigue, slow heartbeat, high triglycerides, dry skin and hair, cold hands and feet, depression, menstrual problems, and memory disturbances. Our goal is to keep metabolism at the most efficient level so that the body can do its work without wasting too much energy as heat.

Where does leptin fit in? It is the master hormone that helps to regulate the thyroid. In times of starvation, leptin levels fall, signaling the thyroid and other hormones to switch into conservation mode. Metabolism slows down but becomes more efficient, body temperature lowers, and vital nutrients are conserved. Leptin resistance distorts the signals that this hormone sends to the thyroid and the rest of your body, and may direct well-fed, even obese individuals into the energy accumulation and fat-storage mode.

There are several tests for thyroid function, but I only use two. One is free T3, which measures blood levels of the unbound form of the most active thyroid hormone. The other is TSH, thyroid stimulating hormone. TSH is the stimulus from the brain that tells the thyroid how much hormone to produce. The bulk of T3 is transported by thyroxine-binding globulin (TBG). Only 0.3 percent of the T3 in the blood is free, but that small percentage is responsible for the many biological actions of thyroid hormone.

The ideal blood level of free T3 is 2.2 to 3.0 pg/mL and, within this range, the lower the level, the better, provided that TSH is within the healthy range of 1.5 to 3.5.

■ BASAL BODY TEMPERATURE

Another way to determine your metabolic rate is to measure your basal body temperature. This reflects your basal metabolism, the amount of energy your body is using when you are at complete rest. An elevated basal temperature is a clear sign that your metabolism is revved up and your thyroid is running on overdrive.

Basal body temperature is best measured upon awakening before you get out of bed and just before you fall asleep at night. It requires a basal thermometer, which is more sensitive than an ordinary thermometer. Digital basal thermometers are most convenient, but any basal thermometer will do. Have the thermometer at your bedside before going to sleep. If it is a glass thermometer, shake it down below 96 degrees the night before. When you awaken, before getting out of bed and while still lying down, take your temperature. Record it, and repeat for at least four to five consecutive days. Go through the same process at night, after lying in bed just before falling asleep. When you are done, remember to prepare the thermometer for your morning reading. A digital thermometer will beep when the temperature has been recorded.

The average basal body temperature is about 97.8 degrees F. The 98.6 degrees you have always been told is normal reflects daytime temperatures, when we are more active. In any case, body temperature varies slightly from one person to the next. What you are looking for are trends and patterns. As the hormonal signals that govern your metabolism become more efficient, your basal temperature will likely go down. This decline will not be dramatic—it may be as little as 0.2 degrees or as much as a full degree—but it will be a very important sign that you are no longer wasting so much energy by generating excess heat. That fuel is instead being used to regenerate your body.

Basal body temperature: 96.8-97.5 degrees F or less optimal (or decline of up to 1 degree F from baseline).

▪ INSULIN-LIKE GROWTH FACTOR-1

Insulin-like growth factor-1 (IGF-1), also called somatomedin-C, is the most reliable test for human growth hormone. Growth hormone is produced in the pituitary gland, released in spurts most abundantly during sleep and exercise. It is a very short-lived hormone and within minutes is broken down in the liver into IGF-1 (so-named because its molecular structure and some of its actions mimic insulin), and remains in the blood for a day or two. Human growth hormone, as its name implies, is partly responsible for growth. Levels build gradually throughout childhood, peak during adolescence, and begin an inexorable decline by the age of twenty. By the time you reach your sixties, you are producing less than 20 percent as much growth hormone as you did in your teens.

For decades, IGF-1 concentrations were only measured in—and growth hormone supplementation was only given to—children of very short stature. Indeed, deficiencies of this hormone during critical stages of development severely retard growth. However, a small study published in 1990 by Daniel Rudman, M.D., in the *New England Journal of Medicine* turned growth hormone into an overnight celebrity. This study, which reported on the effects of six months of growth hormone supplementation in older men, concluded that their improvements in lean muscle mass, body fat, skin thickness, and bone density were "equivalent in magnitude to the changes incurred during ten to twenty years of aging."

Many people, patients and physicians alike, have jumped on the growth hormone bandwagon, regarding it as the fountain of youth and a panacea for aging. I strongly disagree. I maintain that there is a reason why growth hormone and IGF-1 levels fall as we age—and fall most significantly in those who live the longest. In caloric-restricted animals, and those animals genetically modified whose longevity is dramatically increased, IGF-1 levels are almost always much lower than their shorter-lived peers.

IGF-1 is a growth factor. It promotes the growth of cells, and this includes cancer cells. There is a strong correlation between IGF-1 levels and cancer rates. One study showed a fourfold increased risk of prostate cancer in men with the highest IGF-1 levels compared to those with the lowest, and this was independent of baseline PSA levels. Other studies have shown that IGF-1 stimulates the growth of tumors of the breast, lung, and colon and that lowering IGF-1 levels retards cancer growth. Reducing levels of this potent cancer stimulator can only bode well for health and longevity.

IGF-1 levels vary dramatically according to age, but for people who are forty and older, the typical range is from 90 to 360 ng/mL. Your goal should be a downward trend, regardless of your baseline level. I have followed IGF-1 levels in several of my patients, and as they follow the Rosedale Diet, IGF-1 levels decline. Similar to insulin, the goal is optimal sensitivity, not higher levels. At the same time, body fat drops, lean muscle mass increases, and bone density improves. In other words, they achieve the same, in fact higher, benefits that the purveyors of growth hormone offer—without the risks. Improving leptin sensitivity converts energy from cellular replication/reproduction (increased risk of cancer) toward maintenance and repair (increased health and life span).

IGF-1: for ages forty and over, 90 to 360 ng/mL normal; optimal levels not yet determined, reduced "low normal" preferred.

▪ NOREPINEPHRINE

Norepinephrine is a neurotransmitter that facilitates communication in the sympathetic nervous system, which engages during times of stress. This neurotransmitter, along with epinephrine, prepares you to fight or flee from perceived dangers. Your heart rate speeds up and your blood pressure climbs. Glycogen stored in the liver is converted into glucose for anaerobic use, and fatty acids are mobilized for a burst of energy, among many other changes.

Without this crucial reflex it is unlikely that our ancestors could have outrun predators or chased down prey. The problem is that in modern life, most of our stressors do not require fight or flight. For the most part, stress leaves us all revved up with no place to go. When you are under a lot of stress, including the stress of leptin resistance, your sympathetic nervous system goes into overdrive. This takes a toll on the system and can lead to chronically high blood pressure and blood sugar, mental and emotional stress, and increased risk of disease.

The best marker of sympathetic nervous system activity is the blood or urine level of norephinephrine. Normal levels for a blood test are between 250 and 350 pg/mL. How can you keep norepinephrine levels on an even keel? Well, you can learn to relax, avoid responding to stress, and you can lower your leptin levels by increasing your leptin sensitivity. Leptin stimulates the sympathetic nervous system. Leptin resistance is associated with high thyroid, high blood pressure, and elevated blood glucose and fatty acid levels; all are manifestations of sympathetic nervous system activity. The sympathetic nervous system also appears to be the mediator in leptin's effects on bone mass, and is yet another reason to keep tabs on your norepinephrine levels.

Norepinephrine: 250 to 350 pg/mL good, low normal is optimal.

■ HIGHLY SENSITIVE C-REACTIVE PROTEIN (CRP)

Inflammation is part and parcel of your body's response to injury and disease. When cells or tissues are damaged, fibrinogen and other inflammatory compounds that encourage blood clotting are released to stem bleeding. There is a proliferation of immune cells to stave off infection and growth factors to replace damaged cells. After the crisis has passed, levels of these inflammatory compounds should subside.

However, sometimes inflammatory chemicals are elevated in the blood of people who are not overtly sick or injured. This low-grade, chronic inflammation is associated with increased risk of heart disease, diabetes, cancer, autoimmune disorders, and other health problems.

One of the best markers for systemic inflammation is highly sensitive C-reactive protein (CRP), a protein that is produced during inflammation. Studies spearheaded by Paul M. Ridker, M.D., a cardiologist and researcher at Brigham and Women's Hospital and Harvard Medical School, have found that a high level of CRP is a highly accurate predictor of future heart attack; people with the highest levels have up to 4.4 times the risk as those with the lowest levels. CRP is also a very reliable marker for insulin resistance and risk of type 2 diabetes. In a recent study published in *JAMA*, researchers discovered that the women with the highest CRP levels were an astounding 15.7 times more apt to develop type 2 diabetes than those with the lowest levels.

Evidence is also accumulating that inflammation is closely tied to leptin resistance. As body fat increases, CRP levels rise, for the fat cells themselves are a major producer of inflammatory molecules called cytokines. In fact, leptin itself is from the cytokine family. The most significant increases are with central or abdominal obesity, and as you now know, this type of fat deposition is linked to leptin resistance.

Highly sensitive C-reactive protein: less than 1.0 optimal and the lower the better (Note: Request the highly sensitive C-reactive protein test, rather than the standard, less sensitive C-reactive protein test.)

■ TRIGLYCERIDES

Triglyceride is the medical term for fat. Most of the fats we eat, from healthful olive oil to undesirable saturated fats, are in the form of triglycerides. It is also the body's dominant form of stored fat—those love handles and saddlebags are primarily comprised of triglycerides. Triglycerides are ferried around the body by water-soluble chylomicrons, which pick up triglycerides that are absorbed into the bloodstream after a meal, and by very low density lipoproteins (VLDL) that are produced by the liver to mobilize stored fats.

Your triglycerides can be easily measured on a fasting blood test. A level of 50 to 100 mg/dL indicates that you are capable of burning fat efficiently, that your body is not churning excessive amounts of fat into your bloodstream or, more likely than not, a combination of the two A TGL of 100–150 is moderate and over 150 is high, both red flags that you may not be burning fat efficiently. Although they could be an indicator of liver disease, pancreatitis, or low thyroid function, high triglycerides are in most cases a marker of leptin and insulin resistance. They are a clear sign that you are making lots of fat out of your sugar, and that the fats in your blood are not being burned—you are storing fat and burning sugar.

A high triglyceride level is an independent risk factor for heart disease (perhaps because of its association with leptin and insulin). In fact, recent research suggests it is much more predictive of a heart attack than elevated cholesterol.

Although the normal triglycerides range for most labs is up to 150 mg/dL, I think this is too high. While I consider levels up to 125 mg/dL to be acceptable and around 100 mg/dL even better, the level most reflective of optimal leptin sensitivity is under 100 mg/dL. If your triglycerides are elevated, I have good news for you: triglycerides are extremely responsive to the Rosedale Diet. I've had patients whose initial triglyceride levels of 2,000 to 3,000 mg/dL have dropped down into the 200s in a matter of weeks after starting on the program. Cutting back on nonfiber carbohydrates, eating more healthy fats, and, in stubborn cases, taking additional fish oil and niacin supplements work far better than any drug on the market for lowering triglycerides.

Triglycerides: 100 mg/dL optimal; 100 to 135 mg/dL acceptable; 135+ mg/dL high.

■ HOMOCYSTEINE

Homocysteine is a by-product of the metabolism of methionine, an amino acid found in protein. In a process called methylation, homocysteine is rapidly converted into harmless amino acids. However, sometimes the methylation process goes awry, and homocysteine builds up in the blood. This is bad news, for this amino acid is extremely irritating to the arteries. It dampens the production of nitric oxide, which protects the endothelial cells lining the arteries and allows arteries to dilate, and sets the stage for atherosclerosis. Homocysteine also accelerates the oxidation of LDL cholesterol and makes the platelets in the blood stickier, increasing the risk of blood clots that may cause heart attacks or stroke.

If your homocysteine level is elevated, you have more to worry about than heart disease. It also damages neurons in the hippocampus, an area of the brain involved in memory and learning, conferring a threefold elevation in risk of Alzheimer's disease, according to some studies. Methylation is also crucial for DNA repair, so elevations in homocysteine may illuminate underlying problems that may lead to cancer and premature aging.

Most labs consider the normal range to be 5 to 15 umol/L. I suggest you aim for the low end of that range—an ideal level would be no more than 6 umol/L. Some studies have shown a progressive increase in risk of heart attack when homocysteine climbs above 6.3 umol/L. Up to 7 umol/L is acceptable, but when you get over 9 umol/L and especially up toward 13, you can get into trouble.

Early studies suggest that homocysteine and leptin are, if not interactive, then at least coexisting: when homocysteine levels are elevated, so are leptin levels, indicating the presence of leptin resistance. Fortunately, lowering homocysteine levels is relatively easy. Cutting back on coffee and methionine-rich meat will help to some degree, but getting adequate amounts of folic acid, vitamin B12, and vitamin B6 is a sure ticket to lowering homocysteine. The nutrient-rich Rosedale Diet supplies a good portion of your daily vitamin needs, and the supplement program provides the rest. If your homocysteine level does not respond to the suggested levels of these B-complex vitamins, you likely have a genetic variation that requires more intense supplementation. Simply increase your B-vitamin intake, and your homocysteine level will drop.

The recommended levels of the homocysteine-lowering vitamins are 800 micrograms of folic acid, 150 micrograms of vitamin B12, and 75 milligrams of vitamin B6. (If you are older than age 55, consider increasing your vitamin B12 intake up to 1,000 micrograms to compensate for age-associated declines in vitamin B12 absorption.) If your homocysteine level is high, double your folic acid intake and increase your vitamin B12 to 1,000 micrograms. If that doesn't do the trick, you can go as high as 5,000 micrograms of folic acid and 2,500 micrograms of vitamin B12 and add 1,000 milligrams of trimethylglycine (TMG, sometimes called betaine), which also facilitates the methylation process. These vitamins are quite safe, but I wouldn't go too high on vitamin B6, for prolonged use of very high doses has been implicated in nerve damage.

Homocysteine: less than 6 umol/L optimal; Up to 8 umol/L acceptable; over 9 umol/L high; over 13umol/L very high.

■ BUN (BLOOD UREA NITROGEN)

BUN is a common blood test that measures for urea nitrogen, a product of protein metabolism. When you eat protein, it is broken down into nitrogen-containing amino acids. The nitrogen is removed and combined with other molecules to produce urea, which eventually makes its way to the kidneys where it is eliminated in the urine. If kidney function is compromised, BUN levels rise above the normal range of 7 to 25 mg/dL.

Although this test is routinely used to evaluate kidney function, I use it to monitor my patients' protein intake. The average BUN hovers around 18–22 mg/dL. If a person is eating too much protein, his or her BUN will be in the upper range of normal. A common mistake people make as they adjust to the Rosedale Diet is eating too much protein. This is easy to do since fat and protein are often found in the same foods, and many assume that if they're following other low carb/high-fat diets, they're okay. (In reality, many "high-fat diets" such as the Atkins diet are really high-protein diets.) A key principle of the Rosedale Diet is moderate, not high, intake of protein. Regular monitoring of BUN can help ensure dietary compliance.

BUN: 17 mg/dL optimal; up to 21 mg/dL acceptable; more than 21 mg/dL high.

▪ CREATININE

Creatinine is a marker of kidney function. It is a breakdown product of creatine, a constituent of muscle tissue. When the kidneys are functioning properly, creatinine is excreted at a constant rate. If the kidneys are diseased or damaged, however, excretion becomes less efficient, and creatinine builds up in the blood.

A primary contributor to kidney damage is diabetes, and as the cells become more sensitive to insulin and blood glucose levels normalize on the Rosedale Diet, creatinine levels often go down. The ideal range for creatinine is 0.7 to 1.0 mg/dL. (Levels vary among individuals depending on muscle mass; creatinine is generally higher in men than in women.) Although up to 1.4 mg/dL is considered within normal limits, levels of 1.3 or 1.4 mg/dL are indicative of borderline kidney function. When levels are over 1.4 mg/dL, you are looking at partial kidney failure.

Creatinine: 0.7 to 1.0 mg/dL optimal; 1.1 mg/dL to 1.2 mg/dL acceptable; 1.3 to 1.4 mg/dL borderline high; 1.4 mg/dL and above high.

▪ URIC ACID

Uric acid is a breakdown product of the metabolism of purines, which are produced in the body (they are the building blocks of DNA and RNA) and are found in the diet most abundantly in fish, shellfish, turkey, and some types of meat. When there is an overproduction of uric acid or an inability of the kidneys to excrete it, uric acid levels build up in the blood.

Until recently, elevated levels of uric acid were associated only with gout. Chronically high concentrations of uric acid can collect in the tissues and form sharp crystals in the joint fluid, causing the intense pain and swelling characteristic of gout. However, research over the past few years has determined that high levels of uric acid are also found in individuals with high blood pressure, elevated cholesterol, diabetes, and weight problems—all signs and symptoms of leptin and insulin resistance. In one large study, increased uric acid levels were found to be highly predictive of increased risk of death from heart attack or stroke.

You would do well to keep your uric acid level within the normal range of 3 to 7 mg/dL. And no, you don't have to curtail your intake of purine-rich foods, which has been recommended to patients with gout for years. The Rosedale Diet is a much surer path to lowering uric acid levels than the hopelessly outdated low-purine diet.

Uric acid: 3 to 7 mg/dL normal; more than 7 mg/dl high.

▪ LIVER ENZYMES (ALKALINE PHOSPHATASE, ALT, AND AST)

In addition to its roles in detoxification and digestion, the liver plays multiple roles in metabolism. It stores glucose as glycogen, packages fats for storage and transportation, synthesizes proteins, and helps regulate blood sugar. Therefore, we like to keep an eye on how the liver is doing in the Rosedale Diet.

A number of blood tests monitor liver function. These include tests of certain enzymes, which are produced by all tissues in the body but are most concentrated in liver and muscle cells. Enzymes are released into the bloodstream when these tissues are damaged or diseased. Minor elevations in liver enzymes are no cause for concern unless they remain elevated on repeated tests. Commonly tested liver enzymes include alkaline phosphatase, or ALP; ALT, also called SGPT; and AST, sometimes referred to as SGOT.

Liver enzymes: alkaline phosphatase (ALP) 44 to 147 IU/l normal; ALT (SGPT) 5 to 30 IU/l normal; AST (SGOT) 10 to 34 IU/l normal.

■ CHOLESTEROL (TOTAL, HDL, LDL, AND SMALL, DENSE LDL)

The quest to lower cholesterol has reached epidemic proportions in this country. More than 15 million Americans take drugs to lower their cholesterol, and public health officials are urging another 25 million to jump on the bandwagon. I think they're misguided, and I'd like to tell you why. Cholesterol is an essential compound that is required in the production of steroid hormones such as testosterone and estrogen. It is also a key structural component of every cellular membrane and is involved in the synthesis of vitamin D and bile, which is required for the digestion of fats. You've probably heard about "good" cholesterol and "bad" cholesterol. The truth is, there's no such thing. Cholesterol is just cholesterol. It is a cholesterol molecule's transport vehicle that makes it more or less problematic.

These transport vehicles are water-soluble proteins called lipoproteins. High density lipoprotein (HDL) is the so-called good cholesterol. This large carrier shuttles excess cholesterol to the liver where it is recycled (because it is so important) or excreted in the bile. Low density lipoprotein (LDL) is the "bad" one by virtue of its smaller size, and the smaller it is the more damaging it can be. Although many doctors are unaware of it, LDL comes in more than one form. The most harmful of all is small, dense LDL, for its small size enables it to slip into and damage the endothelium, or lining of the arteries—an important step in atherosclerosis.

A fasting blood test will measure levels of total cholesterol, HDL, LDL and, if specifically required, small, dense LDL and other subfractions. LDL particle size including small dense LDL is done by certain specialty labs. Optimal levels for cholesterol are considered to be less than 200 mg/dL for total cholesterol, less than 100 mg/dL for LDL, more than 40 mg/dL for HDL, and less than 90 mg/dL for apo B. But frankly, I pay little attention to my patients' cholesterol levels. Only when a patient presents with a level in the high 300s or 400s mg/dL (almost always caused by an underlying genetic defect predisposition) will I be very concerned. I do not believe that a high cholesterol level is nearly as important as the medical profession has brainwashed us into believing. It is merely a symptom of a larger underlying problem. It is the metabolic hormones that regulate its amount and particle size that are much more important.

Cholesterol levels are really a reflection of how much your body needs to manufacture to repair damage and make steroid hormones. If you have leptin and insulin resistance, you're going to need more cholesterol, and you're going to have lower HDL cholesterol, and higher LDL, particularly small, dense LDL. When you correct the underlying hormonal problems and fat burning processes by following the Rosedale Diet, abnormalities in cholesterol will also be corrected. Total cholesterol will go down and, more important, protective HDL will rise while levels of the most dangerous small, dense LDL cholesterol will go down.

Cholesterol: As far as I'm concerned, this test is highly overrated, and that only people with extremely high cholesterol (over 300) should worry about total cholesterol. I believe that what type of cholesterol you have is more important: HDL cholesterol higher than 40 mg/dL; a high proportion of large LDL to small dense LDL.

chapter eleven

Getting Healthy with the Rosedale Diet

▪ HEART DISEASE

Heart disease is the number one killer of both men and women in the United States. Although the incidence of heart disease had been on the decline since the 1960s, it is beginning to creep up again. Since heart disease is so closely linked to obesity and diabetes, this is not surprising.

I consider the high incidence of heart disease to be a "man-made" problem that is caused by metabolic malfunction, not an inevitable disease of aging. It ought to be a rare disease. Due to its close connection to obesity, leptin is also an obvious culprit in heart disease. Leptin resistance is also an *independent* risk factor for cardiovascular disease, meaning that in and of itself, it can directly and negatively affect your heart and arteries. Restoring leptin sensitivity will go a long way in greatly reducing the risk of heart disease and extending your life.

- ▪ Carrying excess fat around your waist and abdomen (having an apple-shaped body), a result of and a telltale sign of leptin resistance, can put a severe strain on your heart, and increases your risk of heart attack.

- Leptin resistance increases the risk (and can be a primary cause) of insulin resistance, which also increases the risk of heart disease.
- Leptin resistance can activate the fight-or-flight response, causing blood vessels to constrict, increasing blood pressure and putting extra strain on the heart, and increasing the risk of stroke.
- Leptin resistance can cause blood vessels to go into spasm, a lesser-known cause of heart attack.
- Elevated leptin levels can promote the formation of blood clots, which increases the risk of heart attack (when a clot interferes with the blood flow to the heart) and stroke (when a clot interferes with the blood flow to the brain).
- Elevated leptin increases the production of chemicals that trigger inflammation, which can promote the formation of plaque, the cellular debris that forms in the lining of the arteries, impairing the flow of blood.
- Leptin resistance confuses your body about where to put calcium. Instead of putting calcium in your bones, you will end up putting it in your arteries. You will simultaneously get both heart disease and osteoporosis.
- Elevated leptin can cause a thickening in the endothelium, the very thin inner lining of the artery. This causes the artery to be less flexible with each heartbeat, raising blood pressure and promoting clots. The endothelium is a very important part of your circulatory system: It produces its own array of hormones to regulate its own blood flow. Injury to the endothelium is a main trigger of inflammation that results in plaque. Leptin resistance also may impair the ability of the endothelium to burn fat, thereby increasing fatty deposits in the artery.

The Standard Treatment

The standard medical treatment for heart disease is a high carbohydrate–low fat diet usually combined with prescription medicine to lower cholesterol. To me, this approach is backward. The medical fixation on lowering cholesterol reflects the typical "treat the symptom, not the underlying cause" approach that is not only ineffective, but in the long run, can be harmful. In recent years, statin drugs (Lipitor, Mevacor, Pravachol, and Zocor) used to lower cholesterol have become among the most widely prescribed drugs in the world. Statin drugs, however, are not without significant side effects. For example, statin drugs can deplete the body of CoQ10, which is essential for providing energy to the cells of the body, especially heart cells that need lots of energy. CoQ10 depletion can result in muscle damage often associated with aches and pains (a common side effect of "statin" drugs). Since your heart is basically a muscle, it is probably getting damaged also, impairing its ability to pump blood and increasing the risk of congestive heart failure. In other words, over time, these drugs can weaken the heart and impair its major function. Sure, in the short run, they may lower cholesterol, but in the long run, they can kill you.

For all the "cholesterol causes heart disease" hype, it might surprise you to learn that cholesterol has never even been proven to cause heart disease. Even if high cholesterol were slightly correlated with heart disease, correlation and cause should never be confused—something else could be causing both. Statin drugs inhibit cholesterol production, but they don't get to the root cause of the overproduction of cholesterol: Something is signaling the liver to produce more cholesterol.

Symptoms are the way your body has learned over the eons to deal with a disease. Extra cholesterol is being manufactured by the liver because it's getting instructions to do so, but why? The importance of elevated cholesterol is not that you have extra cholesterol, it's the fact that your liver is getting a message to make it. You have to know why, and you have to fix the *why*. The *why* could be that the liver is being smothered by too much fat because of leptin resistance and cannot then get the proper instructions from insulin. It could also be that your body, inflamed due to damage, is trying to repair that damage. New cells have to be manufactured to replace the damaged ones, and no cell can be made without cholesterol. What needs to be done is to reduce the damage and correct the instructions being given to the liver, not impair the body's capacity to repair itself.

Cholesterol is also the precursor to manufacture any of the important steroid hormones such as testosterone, progesterone, estrogen, and cortisone. Far from being a villain, cholesterol is required for life. Even though oxygen can "oxidize" you and form dangerous free radicals, no one would ever suggest that you stop breathing! Oxygen is required to keep you alive. So, too, is cholesterol. No life on earth can be made without it.

Interestingly, it has recently been shown that "statin" drugs might offer benefits not by lowering cholesterol, but by reducing inflammation, and perhaps in spite of lowering cholesterol. Once again, it's important to get the root cause of the inflammation, not the body's response to it. There are a number of factors that can inflame your blood vessels and your heart, such as having elevated glucose, leptin, or insulin levels. Following the Rosedale Diet will help solve these problems permanently and go a long way in reversing and preventing heart disease. Within a matter of weeks, you will increase blood flow to your heart and brain (and the rest of your body!) and you will start burning fat in your arteries as well as everywhere else. You don't need to take drugs for the rest of your life to keep your heart healthy.

The Rosedale Rx

If you have been diagnosed with heart or blood vessel disease, you should follow the Rosedale Diet Supplement Plan Plus. I recommend that patients with heart disease add the following supplements to what they are already taking.

Extra CoQ10. CoQ10 is included in the Rosedale Diet Supplement Plan. My patients with congestive heart failure take 200 milligrams levated ferritin (too much iron in your blood) can cause inflammation and hurt your heart. Your doctor should check your ferritin levels at your annual physical. If you have high ferritin levels, you can usually bring them down to normal by periodically donating blood to a blood bank. By doing so, you're helping yourself and you're helping others.

three times daily for a total of 600 milligrams. CoQ10 improves your heart's ability to pump blood, which is fundamental to your survival.

Extra Arginine. Arginine is included in the Rosedale Diet Supplement Plan. It should be taken in higher doses by people with heart disease. I prescribe up to 6 grams daily for my patients with heart disease.

Vinpocetine. Vinpocetine is not included in the Rosedale Diet Supplement Plan. Vinpocetine is an extract of the periwinkle plant, *Vinca minor,* the same plant that has given us potent cancer treatments for childhood leukemia. For more than two decades, vinpocetine has been used in Europe and Japan to treat stroke victims and people suffering from dementia due to impaired blood circulation to the brain. Vinpocetine dilates arteries and improves blood flow. It is also a potent antioxidant.

Take one 10-milligram capsule twice daily.

If you have elevated homocysteine, I recommend the following additional supplements.

Vitamin B12. For best absorption, use the sublingual form (a tablet that melts under the tongue) Take one 1-milligram tablet daily.

Trimethylglycine (TMG). This supplement can help convert harmful homocysteine into harmless by-products. Take one 250-milligram tablet twice daily. (Some people may need to go up to 1,000 milligrams daily to achieve the desired result.)

Folic Acid. This B-vitamin helps reduce homocysteine levels. Take one 400-microgram tablet daily.

■ DIABETES

The increased incidence in diabetes is as shocking as it is alarming. This is a disease that should be very rare, yet it is commonplace, even among children, and rapidly escalating. At one time, type 2 diabetes was called senile diabetes, a reflection of the fact that it usually did not affect people until they were well into their late decades. As more and more middle-age people began to develop this disease, the name was changed to adult-onset diabetes (no one middle-aged wants to be called senile!). Given the fact that so many children are now getting adult-onset diabetes, medicine has once again stuck a name onto a so-called new disease—MODY, Maturity-Onset Diabetes of the Young. This is a prime example of how the so-called diseases of aging are not related solely to chronological age, but to overall health.

Type 1 diabetes (also called juvenile diabetes) is a result of too little insulin, the hormone that is produced in response to rising blood glucose or sugar levels. Without enough insulin, blood sugar levels can climb dangerously high, leading to organ damage and death. Type 2 diabetes (discussed in the paragraph above) is an entirely different story and accounts for about 95 percent of all cases of adult diabetes. Type 2 diabetes is characterized by a condition called insulin resistance, which occurs when the cells of the body are constantly exposed to high levels of insulin. Plenty of insulin is being made, but cells have become desensitized. In the case of type 2 diabetes, the cause is more closely linked to a failure in cellular communication, that is, how well your cells can "listen" to insulin and leptin, than your age.

When your cells become resistant to insulin, the receptors on cell membranes no longer "hear" the signals from insulin. This can cause catastrophic health problems down the road, including blood lipid abnormalities, high blood pressure, heart disease, and even cancer.

Insulin resistance often goes hand in hand with elevated leptin levels and leptin resistance, and both conditions are linked to eating too much of the wrong food. Lower your leptin levels and your insulin problems will greatly improve.

- Leptin resistance results in deep pockets of fat in the waist and abdomen which "smother" the liver from receiving proper hormonal signals, a very important one being from insulin. When your liver becomes insulin resistant, it will make too much sugar, contributing to insulin resistance and diabetes.
- Elevated leptin also increases fight-or-flight mode, which boosts blood glucose levels and production of cortisol (stress hormone) by the adrenal glands, which causes blood glucose levels to soar even higher.

The Standard Treatment

The current strategy for treating either form of diabetes is to use drugs to control blood sugar levels. I think that this approach is backward: Contrary to what everyone is taught, including your doctor, diabetes is not a disease of blood sugar, it is a disease of insulin signaling. As the warden famously said to Paul Newman in the movie *Cool Hand Luke*, "What we have here is a failure to communicate." Diabetes is perhaps the quintessential disease of cellular miscommunication. Type 2 diabetes should more appropriately be called insulin resistant diabetes; the body is not effectively using the insulin it produces. Once again, the real solution is to treat the underlying cause of the problem, not the symptom.

The conventional treatment of diabetes is typical of what happens when you treat symptoms instead of the underlying disease. Drugs used to treat diabetes most often cause more problems down the road than they help. There is only one standard drug that helps to improve insulin sensitivity somewhat: metformin, sold under the brand name Glucophage. For decades, most drugs used to treat diabetes lowered blood sugar by "whipping" your pancreas to produce even more insulin, causing insulin resistance to worsen and further damaging the already stressed cells that manufacture insulin (islet cells of the pancreas). Other drugs (such as pioglitazone, sold under the brand name Actos, and rosiglitazone maleate, sold under the brand name of Avandia) purported to restore insulin sensitivity work by lowering blood sugar levels in one of the worst possible ways—they create new fat cells to store the excess sugar. If you weren't obese to begin with, once you've been taking these drugs for a while, you will be. Sure, you lower blood sugar temporarily, but at a steep price. Being fatter will only increase your risk of many diseases down the road, including diabetes.

Diabetes is mostly a nutritional disease and must be treated as such. The real "cure" for diabetes is to eat a diet that promotes insulin and leptin sensitivity.

The Rosedale Rx

The good news is that type 2 diabetes (insulin resistant diabetes) can not only be improved, but can often be completely reversed. Even type 1 diabetes can be greatly helped by following my program. With proper insulin sensitivity, a relatively small amount of insulin is necessary to communicate its vital messages of what to do with energy. As long as the diabetes—or the drugs used to treat diabetes—have not completely destroyed the ability of the pancreas to produce insulin, following the Rosedale Diet will in most cases reverse the disease. You will likely need to lower your dose of many medications, including high blood pressure medications and insulin, and many of you will be able to go off them altogether. *This should be done only under your doctor's supervision.* Even if your pancreas is not producing any insulin and you must always take insulin, you can still benefit from my program. The diet and supplement regimen will greatly improve your insulin sensitivity so that you can manage on less insulin, which reduces your risk of developing complications caused by excess insulin. In addition, your blood sugar will be on much less of a roller coaster, with fewer low sugar episodes.

Moderate exercise is also a wonderful way to burn off sugar, as long as you don't overdo it and overstress your body (which can raise blood sugar levels).

If you have been diagnosed with diabetes, you should follow the Rosedale Diet Supplement Plan Plus. I recommend that patients with diabetes take additional amounts of the following supplements:

Vanadyl Sulfate. Take 20 milligrams three times daily for a total of 60 milligrams until blood sugar is under better control. Discontinue if sugar goes low after stopping your other diabetic medications.

Extra Thiamine. Take one 50-milligram capsule twice daily.

Extra Alpha Lipoic Acid. Take one 200-milligram capsule three times daily for a total of 600 milligrams daily. (Always take lipoic acid with food; it's easier on the stomach.)

■ OSTEOPOROSIS

If you follow the Rosedale Diet, I can promise several things. You will lose unwanted fat; that's a given. Once you stop burning so much sugar and storing fat, you will burn up the excess fat off your body, your blood sugar will lower and you will trim down. And you may be surprised to learn that if you have osteoporosis, this too will be vastly improved. In fact, not only will you stop losing bone, you will begin to rebuild bone.

Osteoporosis is a disease characterized by the thinning of bone, which makes it more vulnerable to fracture. What does leptin have to do with your bones? Everything! Recent studies have shown that leptin may be the most important factor of all in controlling bone formation. Your bones are constantly being broken down and rebuilt so that you have supple, fresh new bones to support your body. It may surprise you to know that estrogen, and all of the drugs used to protect bone density (such as Fosamax) do not even work by promoting the formation of bone. These drugs can only reduce the breakdown of bone, but they don't stimulate the production of new, "young" bone. In the end, they leave you with old, brittle bones. However, it is possible to rebuild your bones so that you have young, strong, supple, pliable bones. How? Keeping your leptin levels low can turn on the repair and maintenance mechanisms in your body that are critical for the growth of new bone. No other pharmaceutical medicine, over-the-counter supplement, or exercise can stimulate the formation of new bone as well as simply lowering your leptin levels!

One of the hallmarks of aging is a reduction in lean body mass. That means you begin to lose muscle and bone. If you are a sugar burner, you accelerate that process: Your body is adapted to burning sugar even when you're not eating, so you're going to burn sugar from your lean body mass and your protein stores, and that's going to be muscle and **bone.**

If you're burning the protein in your bones for sugar, your bones are going to be weaker. Without enough bone protein, calcium has nothing to cling to. I often use the analogy of a house to explain bone strength. What keeps a house standing upright? The frame of the house is the most critical part of any home. If your house has a weak frame, it will eventually crumble. In bone, the equivalent of the frame of the house is its underlying protein matrix (the same protein you burn when you are a sugar burner). Calcium gives the bone rigidity, but not so much strength. Bone density and bone strength are not the same. If you are losing bone because you are a sugar burner, taking calcium supplements is not going to make a bit of difference for bone strength. It can be detrimental to your health in other ways. In fact, bones are somewhat of a wastebasket for calcium because too much of it can be harmful.

Although you need some calcium to live, too much calcium can be dangerous, disrupting cellular communication. You could consider it to be a hormone inside your cells. Just as having too much leptin can be unhealthy, so can too much calcium. Much of the energy in running the body is spent on keeping calcium out of your cells. Here's why maintaining the right amount of calcium is so important. When a hormone hits a cell to tell it what to do, its message must be relayed to the cell's library of information—its genes and chromosomes. The hormone doesn't usually go right to the gene; its first stop is usually to a receptor on the cell membrane, which surrounds the cell, or the nuclear membrane. The message from that hormone must then be transferred to the gene. This process almost always involves calcium. When a hormone hits a cell, it allows a trickle of calcium "messengers" into the cell to tell the cell that a hormone just made contact. If there is too much calcium, calcium can disrupt all cellular communication. Trying to pass a message from a hormone to a gene in a high calcium environment would be like trying to carry on a conversation with a friend during a rock concert—you may hear a muffled sound over the loud music, but you can't make out what is being said. Studies have even shown that having higher blood calcium levels, though even in the so-called normal range, can increase your risk of premature death.

Ironically, taking high amounts of calcium to stem bone loss and rebuild bone can weaken your bones by making it more difficult for your cells to keep unwanted calcium from entering inside the cell, where they can actually disrupt the hormone signals required to manufacture bone—including those from leptin and insulin.

How much calcium do we need? On the Rosedale Diet, you can get about 500–700 milligrams of calcium daily just from eating nuts and vegetables, which is all you need to maintain bone health if your hormones are working properly. Anything more than that runs the risk of causing a breakdown in cellular communication. When your cells cannot hear where to put the calcium that you are taking, some might end up in your bones, but much of it may end up in very wrong places, such as your arteries, resulting in arterial calcification, or hardening, of the arteries.

It is far better to support bone strength by maintaining the protein matrix. The manufacture of the protein matrix is dependent on vitamin K and hormones such as leptin; calcium has little to do with it. Calcium is like the brick used to build a house. You can't build a house by just dumping a bunch of bricks on a lot and hoping they will fall into place. You need to know what to do with them. That goes back to cellular communication, which can be disrupted by too much calcium.

Bone loss is not just a woman's problem. Testosterone is critical for all protein-building, including the protein matrix in bone for both men and women. But if men have too much fat on their bodies, as happens in leptin resistance, they may produce excess amounts of an enzyme called aromatase, which is manufactured in fat cells. This increases the conversion of testosterone into estrogen. Bottom line: When you disrupt the intricate and very exact hormonal symphony that allows any life-form to exist and to live, it starts messing up everything.

What about exercise? Exercise does tend to increase bone strength, but only if the hormonal milieu is correct, that is, only if the bones are insulin sensitive and leptin sensitive. In order to have strong bones, you need to first restore leptin and insulin sensitivity.

The Rosedale Rx

I recommend only one additional supplement for patients who have been diagnosed with, or are at risk for, osteoporosis.

Vitamin K. Vitamin K is essential for the production of GLA proteins, which comprise the protein matrix in bone. It is found in leafy green vegetables, but you may not be able to get enough through diet or your multivitamin alone. I prescribe extra vitamin K to patients who are concerned about developing osteoporosis or who are already showing signs of bone loss. Vitamin K is available in an oil-based supplement that is administered by dropper. (Check the bottle to see how many milligrams of vitamin K are in each dropperful.) To prevent osteoporosis, take 2 milligrams of vitamin K daily. If you already have osteoporosis, take 8 milligrams of vitamin K daily.

▪ ARTHRITIS

Although most patients come to my clinic because they want to lose weight, or are seeking a nutritional approach to treat diabetes, once they begin the Rosedale Diet they are surprised by its wonderful "side benefits." This often includes a remarkable reduction in arthritic-related joint pain. Patients frequently tell me that their previously chronic joint pain is much improved after following my diet. Many are able to stop taking anti-inflammatory pain medication. For example, I recently saw a patient who complained of severe pain in his right arm due to bursitis. It was so painful that he could no longer play tennis, a game that he loved. After a few weeks on the diet, however, much to his delight, the pain had vanished and he could lift his right arm without any discomfort. He is back on the tennis court.

What is the relationship between joint pain and leptin?

The answer has more to do with the relationship between leptin and all diseases than just about arthritis. As I've said earlier, I believe that even though the medical community has given each disease a name based on the specific anatomical part that is affected and is visible to the naked eye, the underpinnings of that disease are cellular and bio-chemical. As such, each disease does not originate at a particular anatomical location, but from a general problem in cellular communi-cation. In the case of arthritis—whether it's osteoarthritis (so-called wear-and-tear arthritis) or rheumatoid arthritis (due to an overactive im-mune system)—the disease occurs as a result of excessive inflammatory signals, and those excessive inflammatory signals are going to be medi-ated, as with any signals, by hormones.

Anytime you feel pain, it is due to inflammation of something, somewhere in your body. Whether it's inflammation of a nerve or in-flammation of a joint, pain is being mediated by hormonal signals. We think of pain as coming from nerves, but nerves are merely a way to telegraph messages via hormones called neurotransmitters. Whatever is going on in your body, it always relates back to hormones and cellular communication, without exception. If you're stabbed by a knife, the reason it hurts is because your cells are telling you that you are in dan-ger. The reason the wound might kill you is because of a disruption in cellular communication. If you bleed too much, your cells won't get the nourishment they need to talk to one another. For instance, your heart cells may no longer be able to communicate with one another and therefore your heart may stop beating. In the case of arthritis, even though we see it and feel it in the joint, what is causing that inflamma-tion can be triggered or amplified by signals from elsewhere in the body.

All cellular miscommunication either originates from or at the very least is aggravated by leptin and insulin resistance. An increase in leptin and/or insulin levels will amplify whatever pain you are experiencing, and that includes joint pain.

Joint diseases fall into two categories: wear-and-tear and autoimmune. Wear-and-tear arthritis—osteoarthritis and bursitis—is due to overuse.

The mechanism behind autoimmune joint diseases is less obvious. In an autoimmune disease, for reasons that are not fully understood, the body's own immune system attacks cells in a particular organ system. In the case of rheumatoid arthritis, immune cells attack cells in the joint. Why a particular body part becomes targeted by the immune system is pretty much anybody's guess, but the latest theories focus on a concept called molecular mimicry. All life-forms mimic each other; in other words, they are very similar. We have to eat life to maintain our own. In some cases, food is not completely digested in the gut, and bigger protein molecules end up getting through the gut lining into the bloodstream. These larger molecules may mimic some of our body's molecules. If amino acid sequences in these little foreign protein fragments closely resemble the protein composition of particular body parts, such as joints, these molecules are deemed to be foreign particles by the immune system and the immune system will attack them. For example, the immune cells may start to attack joints as well. Wheat and dairy are prime culprits—they contain protein components similar to human tissue.

Or if the foreign protein particles in food are similar to the islet cells in the pancreas, immune cells will attack them and they will stop making insulin, which can lead to type 1 or insulin dependent diabetes. If you have mild inflammation of your gut (inflammatory bowel disease), even so mild that you don't know anything is wrong, inflammatory hormones are released and transmitted through the blood that can aggravate inflammation elsewhere in your body, such as your joints.

What could cause a glitch in digestion that could result in poorly digested proteins? Frequent use of antacids can interfere with the proper digestion of protein. The overuse of antibiotics, which kills off beneficial bacteria in the gut that aid in digestion and keep your gut cells healthy, might let incompletely digested proteins to be absorbed. High leptin levels stimulate the production of inflammatory hormones by cells (T cells) of the immune system. A high leptin level will magnify and multiply your weak points throughout your body. For example, if you have a slightly inflamed joint in your shoulder or your knee, and if your leptin or insulin is high, it will cause you significantly more discomfort than if your leptin levels are at healthy levels. This is how, by following the Rosedale Diet and keeping leptin levels low, many symptoms due to excess inflammation (called diseases by the medical establishment) including arthritis, allergies, and even cardiovascular disease are greatly reduced.

The Rosedale Rx

Within a few weeks of following the Rosedale Diet Supplement Plan, most people find that their inflammatory symptoms, including those of arthritis, are significantly better. Some people who are affected more severely, however, may need additional help to relieve symptoms. I recommend two supplements to my patients that are shown to reduce the pain and inflammation associated with either form of arthritis. Neither supplement is included in the Rosedale Diet Supplement Plan.

Glucosamine. Glucosamine is a natural constituent of cartilage, the substance that lines the joints. It has been widely touted as one of the supplements in the so-called "arthritis cure." Although it's not a cure for arthritis, it can relieve some of the discomfort. I recommend taking 500 milligrams of glucosamine twice a day if necessary (but generally not more).

Cetyl Myristoleate. The supplement is lesser-known than glucosamine, but is also good for symptomatic relief. Cetyl myristoleate is derived from mistletoe and is an anti-inflammatory. Take one 500-milligram capsule daily.

Afterword

Now that you have been following the Rosedale Diet, based on the experiences of my patients, I can make the following assumptions. First, you are losing excess weight, quickly and safely. Second, you are no longer walking around hungry. You feel satisfied. And third, you feel happier and more energized than you have in years. You are undoubtedly thrilled that you are losing fat, and it's great to see your waistline begin to shrink and your body become more defined, but you are noticing other good things too. Many of you are mentally sharper, sleeping better, and in general, feeling better.

Everybody—myself included—wants to look in the mirror and feel good about what they see. But as I tell my patients, it's what you *don't* see that is even more important. You don't see your cells becoming sensitive to leptin's messages, your glucose levels falling, your insulin levels normalizing, or the excess fat deposits disappearing from your arteries. Yet all these positive things are happening. In other words, you are regaining your health and vitality, and that is what the Rosedale Diet is all about.

I encourage you to stay on the Rosedale Diet even after you have achieved your weight loss goals. The truth is, I never designed the diet with weight loss in mind. I consider my diet to be the optimal diet that can help you achieve an enhanced and longer life. A wonderful side benefit is that you will be living that life in a well-toned, trim body. The Rosedale Diet is for those who want the best and who want to be the best.

I understand that nobody is perfect, and that there will be times when you may fall off the diet, sometimes for weeks at time. If this happens, I don't want you to think that all is lost. You can always come back to the Rosedale Diet and pick up where you left off. Your body is not static: It is always changing, for better or for worse. With the right tools (that is, the right diet) you can trigger those wonderful repair mechanisms that will keep your body lean, strong, and disease free. My motto is: It's never too late to improve your health. Of course, the longer you are on the diet, the better your results, but there are benefits to be gained at any point in life.

I learn as much from my patients as they learn from me. I would love to hear about your experiences on the Rosedale Diet and how you're doing. Please write me at

Ron Rosedale, M.D.
P.O. Box 370508
Denver, CO 80237-0508

For updates on the Rosedale Diet and information on pending research studies, visit my Web site at www.RosedaleMetabolics.com.

Rosedale Resources

Your 21-Day Food Diary

For the first three weeks on the Rosedale Diet, write down everything you eat, including snacks. Please keep track of your daily intake of protein grams. Make copies of this form and carry it with you for the first 21 days you are following the diet.

Allowable Protein Grams Per Day _____

Date _____   Protein Grams

_____

_____

_____

_____

_____

_____

_____

_____

_____

_____

_____

_____

_____

Total

How Much Protein Should You Eat Every Day?

O n page 207, I list general guidelines on how to estimate how much protein you should eat daily. However, the best method to determine your daily protein requirement and to follow your progress in losing that extra unwanted fat (and, I hope, your increased development of muscle and bone) is to purchase a home body fat analyzer. They are available at many department stores and have become quite accurate and much more affordable in recent years. Simply follow the directions to determine your percentage of fat composition and pounds of fat. There should also be directions to determine your lean mass. If not, it is quite easy. Subtract your fat weight in pounds from your total weight to obtain a close approximation of your lean body mass in pounds. Then, to obtain your daily protein requirement in grams, simply divide your lean body mass in half. Add approximately 10 grams of protein to your total if you are a heavy exerciser. (Remember to spread out your protein intake throughout the day for most efficient utilization.) I have used a professional body fat analyzer made by the Tanita corporation in my office for many years and have been very pleased with its performance. They also produce a home version that is quite affordable, and many of my patients who own one have been happy with it. To obtain more information on their products, you can call them at 800-9-TANITA. Other body fat analyzers are also available in stores and may be quite acceptable.

For those of you who do not wish to purchase a body fat analyzer, the following formulas work quite well to determine protein needs. However, please be aware that for those of you who have put on a significant amount of weight in your hips (a pear shape), and for those women who are not overweight and have very narrow hips, the results may not be as accurate.

▪▪▪ For Women Only:

STEP 1:
Weigh yourself and write down the results.
I weigh _____ lbs.

STEP 2:
Measure your waist size and write down the results.
My waist size is _____ inches.

STEP 3:
Measure your hip size (from the widest point) and write down the results.
My hip size is _____ inches.

STEP 4:
Subtract 6 inches from hips; this equals your *adjusted hip* measurement.
My adjusted hip measurement is _____ inches.

STEP 5:
If your waist is equal to or smaller than your adjusted hip measurement:

To get your daily protein intake in grams simply divide your weight in half.

Weight _____ divided by 2 = _____ daily protein grams

If your waist is larger than your adjusted hip measurement, go to Step 6.

STEP 6:

Subtract your adjusted hips from your waist.

Waist _____ minus adjusted hips _____ = Amount waist is larger than adjusted hips _____

STEP 7:

Multiply the amount your waist is larger than your hips (Answer from question 6) by 7.

_____ × 7 = _____

STEP 8:

Subtract answer from Step 7 from your weight.

Weight _____ minus answer from Step 7 = _____

STEP 9 (YOU'RE ALMOST DONE . . . PROMISE!)

To get your daily total protein intake in grams:

Divide answer from Step 8 by two. _____

Then:

Subtract 5 from that total. (−5) _____

Your Total Daily Protein Intake in Grams _____

If you are diabetic, subtract 5 grams of protein from your final total.

If you are a heavy exerciser, add 10 grams protein to your final total.

···For Men Only:

PROTEIN REQUIREMENT WORKSHEET

STEP 1:
Weigh yourself and write down the results.
I weight _____ lbs.

STEP 2:
Measure your waist size and write down the results.
My waist size is _____ inches.

STEP 3:
Measure your hip size (from the widest point) and write down
the results.
My hip size is _____ inches.

STEP 4:
If your waist is equal to or smaller than your hips:
To get your daily protein intake in grams simply divide your
weight in half.
Weight _____ divided by 2 = _____ daily protein
grams
If your waist is larger than your hips, go to Step 5.

STEP 5:
Subtract your hips from your waist.
Waist _____ minus hip measurement _____ = Amount waist is
larger than hips _____

STEP 6:
Multiply the amount your waist is larger than your hips (answer from
question 5) by 7.
_____ × 7 = _____

STEP 7:
Substract answer from Step 6 from your weight.
Weight _____ minus answer from Step 7 = _____

STEP 8: (YOU'RE ALMOST DONE . . . PROMISE!)
To get your daily total protein intake in grams:
Divide answer from Step 8 in half. _____
Your Total Daily Protein Intake in Grams _____
If you are diabetic, subtract 5 grams of protein from total.
If you are a heavy exerciser add 10 grams protein to total.

Rosedale Diet Recipes

The Rosedale Diet recipes were designed with the help of a friend and colleague, Jena Latham, an herbalist, organic gardener, and private chef who lives in Maui, Hawaii. Her recipes are truly inspired.

■ ■ ■ EGGS "BENEFIT"

This is a healthy, low-carb alternative to an old favorite. Rosemary is a potent antioxidant known to promote circulation to the brain and enhance memory.

SERVES 2

SAUCE

> 3 tablespoons low-fat cream cheese
> ½ teaspoon chopped fresh rosemary
> 1 tablespoon fresh lemon juice
> 1 teaspoon flax oil
> 1 teaspoon avocado oil
> Salt to taste
> Pinch of cayenne
>
> 2 eggs
> 1 ripe avocado
> "Manna from Heaven" bread (see Note and Product Information, page 291), toasted

1. Mix the sauce ingredients in a small bowl with a fork.
2. In a deep skillet, add 2 inches of water, bring to a boil, then turn down to simmer.
3. Crack each egg one at a time into a shallow cup, then gingerly slip each egg into the water, getting very close to the surface. Simmer the eggs for 5 minutes, then remove them with a slotted spoon and drain off excess water.
4. Toast the bread.
5. Slice the avocado in half first, then remove the pit by gently squeezing the avocado.
6. Slice the avocado while in its skin. Remove the avocado meat with your thumbs and place on the toasted bread.
7. Top the bread and avocado with poached eggs and top with sauce.

NOTE: "Manna from Heaven" bread made by the Julienne Bakery is the preferred bread to be used on this diet.

■ ■ ■ CHICKEN SALAD

This luscious salad is loaded with good fat—walnuts, avocado, and olives. Add crispy romaine lettuce and you've got a great-textured, mouthwatering salad.

SERVES 2

DIJON VINAIGRETTE

½ cup extra virgin olive oil

3 tablespoons red wine vinegar

¼ teaspoon Dijon mustard

1 garlic clove

Salt to taste

Stevia powder (or Splenda) to taste

1 boneless, skinless chicken breast

1 small head romaine lettuce, washed and dried

¼ cup chopped walnuts

6 Kalamata olives, halved and pitted

1 ripe avocado, sliced (see page 215)

1. Mix the vinaigrette in a blender.
2. Bring 2 inches of water to a boil in a deep skillet, reduce to simmer, and add the chicken breasts.
3. Simmer for 10 to 15 minutes. Check to see whether the chicken is completely cooked by cutting into the middle of the breast. The meat should be white, not pink, and juices should run clear, not red.
4. In a salad bowl, combine the lettuce, walnuts, olives, and avocado slices.
5. Add half of the dressing to the salad, toss well, and divide between two plates.
6. Slice the chicken diagonally and arrange on top of each salad.
7. Drizzle more dressing on top of the chicken and serve.

▪ ▪ ▪ DILLED SALMON AND FRESH ASPARAGUS

Salmon is a terrific source of beneficial omega-3 fatty acids. The distinct flavor of salmon is well complemented by fresh dill and tart lemon juice. Make an extra portion to be used for Salmon Salad (page 218) tomorrow.

SERVES 2

MARINADE

⅔ cup extra virgin olive oil

⅓ cup fresh chopped dill

¼ cup fresh lemon juice

Pinch of cayenne

¼ teaspoon salt

Pinch of black pepper

2 6-ounce salmon fillets (one is for lunch tomorrow)

¾ pound asparagus (¼ pound is for lunch tomorrow)

1 tablespoon avocado oil

1. Preheat the oven to 400°F.
2. Mix the marinade ingredients in a blender.
3. Place the salmon fillets, skin side up, in a glass baking dish, cover with the marinade, and refrigerate for at least 1 hour.
4. Bake for 5 minutes, turn the fillets over, and bake for 5 more minutes, skin side down. Test for doneness by seeing that the fish flakes easily and is opaque throughout. Save 2 to 3 tablespoons of the cooked sauce to add to tomorrow's salad dressing.
5. Fill a deep skillet with 1½ inches of water, bring to a boil, and drop the asparagus in. Simmer for 5 minutes, drain, drizzle avocado oil on top. Add salt and pepper to taste.

■ ■ ■ NUTOLA

This is a healthy version of granola, which is normally laden with carbs and bad fat. Warm spiced nuts, plump sweet blueberries, and cream are a delectable combination and make a fabulous breakfast or snack.

SERVES 2

    ½ cup sliced almonds
    ½ cup hazelnuts, skinless
    ½ cup cashews
    ½ cup chopped macadamia nuts
    ½ teaspoon cardamom
    1 teaspoon cinnamon
    Pinch of powdered ginger
    1 tablespoon ghee (clarified butter), melted

    1 cup blueberries
    ½ cup cream

1. Preheat the oven to 400°F.
2. Mix the nuts, spices, and ghee in a medium bowl.
3. Spread the nut mixture on baking sheets and roast for 10 to 15 minutes.
4. Serve warm in bowls, topped with ¼ cup blueberries per person and a touch of cream.

■ ■ ■ SALMON SALAD

Always cook extra salmon so that you can enjoy healthy salads like this one.

SERVES 2

BALSAMIC VINAIGRETTE

　　½ cup extra virgin olive oil

　　2 tablespoons balsamic vinegar

　　2 to 3 tablespoons salmon sauce (from Dilled Salmon and Asparagus, page 217)

　　1 tablespoon fresh lemon juice

　　1 tablespoon chopped fresh dill

　　4 cups baby romaine salad greens, washed and dried

　　6 ounces leftover salmon, broken into bite-sized pieces

　　2 tablespoons chopped fresh dill

　　½ red bell pepper, chopped

　　Leftover asparagus, cut into 1-inch pieces

1. Mix the vinaigrette in a blender.
2. Mix the lettuce, salmon, dill, bell pepper, and asparagus in a salad bowl.
3. Pour the dressing on the salad, toss, and serve.

■ ■ ■ BAKED HALIBUT WITH GREEN BEANS

This tart and creamy sauce is the perfect complement to the mild flavor of halibut.

SERVES 2

SAUCE

　　2 to 3 tablespoons capers

　　½ cup extra virgin olive oil

　　¼ cup fresh lemon juice

　　3 tablespoons chopped fresh basil

　　2 tablespoons chopped fresh parsley

　　1 tablespoon homemade mayonnaise (see recipe on page 284)

2 3-ounce halibut fillets

½ pound green beans, ends snipped

1 garlic clove, chopped

2 tablespoons chopped fresh Italian parsley

1 tablespoon fresh lemon juice

1 tablespoon avocado oil

3 tablespoons slivered almonds

1. Mix the sauce in a blender.
2. Preheat the oven to 400°F.
3. Place the halibut in a glass baking dish, pour the sauce over the fish, cover with aluminum foil, and bake for 10 minutes, or until the fish is opaque throughout.
4. Fill a large saucepan one-half full with water, and bring to a boil. Turn down to simmer, add the green beans, and cook for 5 minutes.
5. Drain the beans and toss with the garlic, parsley, lemon juice, avocado oil, and slivered almonds.

▪ ▪ ▪ HARD-BOILED EGGS AND SWISS CHARD

Here's a simple, healthy, and tasty breakfast. Swiss chard is chock-full of healthy antioxidants.

SERVES 2

FLAX DRESSING

3 tablespoons flax oil

½ cup chopped fresh basil

2 tablespoons sesame seeds

1 tablespoon flax seeds

1 teaspoon tamari

Pinch of cinnamon

2 eggs

1 bunch Swiss chard, washed and chopped

1. Mix the flax dressing in a blender.
2. Place the eggs in a small saucepan, cover with cold water, and bring to a boil. Turn down to simmer for 5 minutes.
3. Fill a large saucepan one-third full with water and bring to a boil. Add the chard and turn down to simmer for 5 minutes. Cool the eggs in cold water, peel, and slice in ¼-inch rounds.
4. Drain the chard and split between two plates.
5. Arrange the sliced eggs on top of the chard, and drizzle with dressing.

■ ■ ■ TUNA SALAD

Here's living proof that good fat can taste great!

SERVES 2

> 1 can chunk white tuna packed in water, drained
> ¼ cup chopped cashews
> 2 tablespoons chopped celery
> 2 tablespoons homemade mayonnaise
> 1 tablespoon chopped scallions
> Pinch of cayenne
> Salt to taste
> "Manna from Heaven" Bread (see "Product Information," page 291), thinly sliced and toasted

1. Mix the tuna, cashews, celery, mayonnaise, scallions, cayenne, and salt well with a fork.
2. Serve over toasted Manna bread.

■ ■ ■ LOBSTER TAILS AND SEAWEED SALAD

Are you really on a diet? It's hard to tell when you are enjoying such delicious seafood! The seaweed tastes especially good if you soak it overnight. You can find seal palm at many health food stores and Asian markets.

SERVES 2

3 lobster tails (you can use the extra one for Lobster Salad, page 223, tomorrow)

LOBSTER SAUCE

2 tablespoons fresh lemon juice

1 tablespoon chopped fresh parsley

3 tablespoons ghee (clarified butter), melted

1 tablespoon avocado oil

Pinch of cayenne

Salt to taste

SEAWEED SALAD

1 cup sea palm, well rinsed and soaked overnight

½ red bell pepper, chopped

1 avocado, cut into pieces

¼ cup sesame seeds

2 tablespoons avocado oil

1 tablespoon fresh lemon juice

Dash of tamari

Pinch of cayenne

1. Fill a large saucepan 2 inches high with water and bring to a boil.
2. Mix the lobster sauce in a small saucepan.
3. Rinse the presoaked sea palm well, drain, and place in a bowl with the bell pepper, avocado, sesame seeds, avocado oil, lemon juice, tamari, and cayenne. Mix well.
4. Place the lobster tails in boiling water and simmer for 5 to 7 minutes, or until they turn red.

5. Heat the lobster sauce, pour in small bowls, and serve with the lobster tails and seaweed salad.

■ ■ ■ SMOOTHIE WITH ALMONDS

Blueberries are packed with potent antioxidants, and have been shown to improve learning and memory in laboratory animals. Perhaps the best reason of all to eat them is that they're delicious, especially when combined with almonds.

SERVES 2

2 scoops whey protein powder
1 teaspoon flax oil
¼ cup raw almonds
½ cup frozen blueberries
16 ounces pure water
¼ teaspoon cinnamon

Mix all the ingredients in a blender and serve.

■ ■ ■ LOBSTER SALAD

Don't wait for special occasions to eat lobster. It's light, delicious, and very satisfying.

SERVES 2

Leftover lobster, cut into bite-sized pieces (see Lobster Tails with Seaweed Salad,
    page 222)
1 tablespoon fresh lemon juice
½ cup chopped fresh Italian parsley
¼ cup chopped celery

2 tablespoons homemade mayonnaise

1 shake of Old Bay Seasoning

1 head Bibb lettuce, washed and dried

1. Combine the lobster, lemon juice, parsley, celery, mayonnaise, and Old Bay Seasoning in a bowl.
2. Gently mix and serve over a bed of lettuce.

■ ■ ■ GRILLED TUNA

This sweet and tangy marinade imparts a lovely flavor to fresh tuna. Grilling the fish adds even more depth.

SERVES 2

MARINADE

1 cup orange juice

1 teaspoon orange zest

2 tablespoons tamari

3 tablespoons fresh lime juice

2 6-ounce tuna steaks (one is for Maui Salad, page 226, tomorrow)

½ cucumber

¼ cup chopped walnuts

1 head Bibb lettuce

1 endive, cut into thin rounds

3 tablespoons dulse seaweed (available at health food stores)

TART VINAIGRETTE

½ cup extra virgin olive oil

2 tablespoons fresh lemon juice

2 tablespoons umeboshi plum vinegar

1 tablespoon chopped fresh rosemary

Dash of tamari

Stevia powder to taste

1. Mix the marinade ingredients.
2. Rinse the tuna steaks, pat dry with paper towels, and place in a glass baking dish, skin side up.
3. Pour the marinade over the tuna and refrigerate for 1 hour.
4. Preheat the grill.
5. Roast the walnuts in a cast-iron skillet until they sizzle, and let cool on a large plate.
6. Cut the cucumber in half lengthwise and chop into thin half-moons.
7. Place the lettuce in a salad bowl with the cucumber, walnuts, endive, and dulse.
8. Mix the vinaigrette and toss with the salad just before serving.
9. Grill the tuna for 5 minutes on each side or until done, save one piece for lunch tomorrow, and divide the other into two portions for tonight.

■ ■ ■ AVOCADO AND SMOKED SALMON TOASTS

Serve this for an elegant brunch or afternoon tea! The delicate flavor of avocado paired with savory smoked salmon is quite delicious.

SERVES 2

1 ripe avocado

1 garlic clove, chopped

1 tablespoon fresh lemon juice

1 teaspoon flax oil

¼ cup chopped fresh cilantro

6 ounces smoked salmon

2 pieces "Manna from Heaven" bread

1. Cut the avocado in half, remove the pit and, using your thumbs, remove the avocado from its skin and place in a food processor.
2. Add the garlic to the processor with the lemon juice, flax oil, and cilantro, and blend.

3. Toast the Manna bread, top with the avocado spread first, and then layer the smoked salmon on top.

▪ ▪ ▪ MAUI SALAD

The flavors in this salad will take you away to an exotic paradise.

SERVES 2

LIME VINAIGRETTE

½ cup extra virgin olive oil

3 tablespoons fresh lime juice

1 garlic clove

Pinch of cayenne

2 tablespoons chopped fresh mint

Salt to taste

Stevia powder to taste

1 head romaine lettuce, washed and dried

1 cup arugula, washed and dried

¼ red bell pepper, chopped

¼ yellow bell pepper, chopped

¼ cup chopped macadamia nuts

Leftover tuna, broken into bite-sized pieces (see Grilled Tuna, page 224)

1. Mix the vinaigrette in a blender.
2. Place the romaine, arugula, bell peppers, and macadamia nuts in a salad bowl.
3. Top the salad with the tuna, pour the dressing over, toss well, and serve.

■ ■ ■ GARLIC SHRIMP

Garlic lovers rejoice!

SERVES 2 WITH LEFTOVERS (SAVE SOME FOR SHRIMP WRAP, PAGE 228, TOMORROW)

MARINADE

⅓ cup fresh lime juice

½ cup extra virgin olive oil

10 to 20 garlic cloves

½ cup chopped fresh cilantro

¼ teaspoon red pepper flakes

Salt to taste

1 pound raw shrimp, peeled and deveined

3 tablespoons extra virgin olive oil

4 cups julienned zucchini (use a mandolin if you have one)

1. Mix the marinade in a blender.
2. Place the shrimp in a bowl with the marinade and refrigerate for 1 hour.
3. Sauté the zucchini in olive oil in a heavy skillet.
4. Place the zucchini in a baking dish, cover with aluminum foil, and keep warm in the oven.
5. Add the shrimp and marinade to the skillet and sauté for about 5 minutes, or just until the shrimp begins to turn pink.
6. Pile the zucchini on each plate and spoon the garlic shrimp on top.

■ ■ ■ SOFT-BOILED EGGS SERVED OVER "MANNA FROM HEAVEN" BREAD

Simple yet satisfying

SERVES 2

> 2 eggs
> 2 pieces "Manna from Heaven" bread, toasted
> Salt to taste
> Pinch of cayenne

1. Place the eggs in a saucepan, cover with cold water, bring to a boil, and turn down to simmer for 3 minutes.
2. Cool the eggs in cold water, and remove the shells.
3. Top each piece of Manna bread with an egg. Cut the eggs on top of the toast, so that the yolks seep into the bread.
4. Sprinkle with salt and cayenne.

■ ■ ■ SHRIMP WRAP

This is a quick, yummy lunch—last night's dinner reincarnated.

SERVES 2

> Leftover shrimp cut into ½-inch pieces (see Garlic Shrimp, page 227)
> ½ cup julienned zucchini, left over from last night's dinner
> 2 tablespoons fresh lemon juice
> 3 tablespoons avocado oil
> ¼ cup chopped fresh cilantro
> 1 tablespoon chopped fresh Italian parsley
> Salt to taste
> Pinch of cayenne
> 2 La Tortilla Factory tortillas
> 1 cup shredded romaine lettuce

1. Mix the shrimp, zucchini, lemon juice, avocado oil, cilantro, parsley, salt, and cayenne.
2. Place the tortillas on a cutting board and divide the shrimp mixture between the two.
3. Form the shrimp mixture into a log shape two-thirds toward the bottom of each tortilla.
4. Add the shredded lettuce just above the shrimp.
5. Fold the tortilla from the bottom around the shrimp and continue to roll the tortilla.
6. Slice the shrimp wrap into rounds and serve.

■ ■ ■ MUNG DAL SOUP AND MESCLUN SALAD

The combination of warming spices and filling beans make this a hearty soup for a chilly day. Mung beans are the beans used for bean sprouts, and they are sold at health stores and many supermarkets. Ghee, or clarified butter, is also sold at health food stores. Garam masala is an Indian spice that is available at Asian markets, many gourmet shops, and health food stores.

SERVES 2 WITH LEFTOVERS

MUNG DAL SOUP

1 cup mung beans

3 tablespoons ghee (clarified butter)

2 garlic cloves, chopped

1 teaspoon minced fresh ginger

2½ cups water

Pinch of turmeric

¼ teaspoon garam masala

½ cup chopped fresh parsley

¼ teaspoon salt

Pinch of cayenne

1. Wash the beans well in a colander.
2. Melt the ghee in a large saucepan, add the garlic and ginger, and sauté for 2 minutes.
3. Add the water, beans, turmeric, and garam masala, and simmer for 1 hour.
4. Add the parsley, salt, and cayenne, puree half of the soup, return to the pot, and serve with salad.

MESCLUN SALAD

>2 cups mesclun greens
>1 ripe avocado, peeled and cut in chunks
>½ green apple, thinly sliced
>¼ cup chopped almonds
>2 teaspoons grated Parmesan

BASIL VINAIGRETTE

>½ cup extra virgin olive oil
>2 tablespoons balsamic vinegar
>½ cup chopped fresh basil
>Stevia powder to taste
>Salt to taste

1. Mix the vinaigrette in a blender.
2. Add mesclun greens, avocado, apple, almonds, and Parmesan to a salad bowl.
3. Pour the dressing over the salad. Toss well and serve.

■ ■ ■ SMOOTHIE WITH CASHEWS

An easy and great-tasting breakfast or snack

SERVES 2

>2 scoops whey protein powder
>¼ cup raw cashews

½ cup blueberries

16 ounces water

Pinch of cinnamon

Mix all the ingredients in a blender and serve.

■ ■ ■ GINGERY CHICKEN SOUP

Before refrigeration, spices such as ginger were once used to preserve food. They are rich in antioxidants, which help retard the damaging effects of oxidation. Ginger takes this old-fashioned chicken soup up a notch while helping to keep you healthy.

SERVES 2 WITH LEFTOVERS (SAVE 2 CUPS CHOPPED CHICKEN FOR SPICY CHICKEN SALAD, PAGE 234)

1 medium chicken cut into pieces

3-inch piece of ginger, peeled and chopped

5 garlic cloves, smashed and peeled

4 celery stalks

1 bunch chopped Italian parsley

1 red onion

9 whole cloves

1 bunch chard, washed

1. Wash the chicken and pat dry with paper towels.
2. Place in a large soup pot and cover with 2 quarts water.
3. Bring to a boil and reduce to simmer.
4. Add the ginger, garlic, celery, and parsley.
5. Cut the ends off the onion, cut in half, and stick cloves in each half.
6. Simmer for 2 to 3 hours.
7. Set up a large colander on top of another large pot.
8. Strain the soup and set aside the chicken for tomorrow's lunch.

9. Return the broth to the heat and bring to a boil.
10. Add the chard and reduce to simmer.
11. Simmer for 10 minutes and serve.

■ ■ ■ ROMAINE SALAD

Light and delicious!

SERVES 2

CITRUS VINAIGRETTE

½ cup extra virgin olive oil

2 tablespoons fresh lemon juice

1 tablespoon fresh lime juice

¼ cup fresh chopped mint

Stevia powder (or other sugar substitute) to taste

3 cups baby romaine lettuce, washed and dried

1 celery stalk, chopped

½ yellow bell pepper, cut in strips

1 small head radicchio, washed and sliced

½ cup pecans

1. Mix the vinaigrette in a blender.
2. Put the rest of the ingredients in a salad bowl, add the dressing, toss, and serve.

■ ■ ■ TOFU AND VEGGIES IN LEMON TAHINI SAUCE

This is my favorite quick, easy, and very healthy dish. The best part is that it tastes so delicious!

SERVES 2

½ block firm, organic tofu

2 tablespoons extra virgin olive oil

1 tablespoon tamari

3 chopped scallions

1 cup thinly sliced red cabbage

2 cups broccoli florets

1 cup snow peas

LEMON TAHINI SAUCE

2 to 3 tablespoons avocado oil

1 to 2 tablespoons tahini

3 tablespoons lemon juice

1 tablespoon tamari

Pinch of cayenne

¼ cup fresh chopped basil

Stevia powder to taste

1. Preheat the oven to 400°F.
2. Rinse the tofu and cut into bite-sized pieces. Place in a glass baking dish and toss with olive oil, tamari, and scallions.
3. Put a large pot half-filled with water on to boil.
4. Bake the tofu for approximately 45 minutes.
5. Put the cabbage in the boiling water, turn down to simmer for 5 minutes, add the broccoli, simmer for 3 more minutes, and add the snow peas for 2 more minutes.
6. Mix the lemon tahini sauce in a blender.
7. Strain the veggies and arrange on plates.
8. Top with the tofu and lavish with lemon tahini sauce.

■ ■ ■ SPICY CHICKEN SALAD

Add a little spice to your chicken salad!

SERVES 2

> 2 cups chicken from Gingery Chicken Soup (page 231), cut into bite sized pieces
> 1 celery stalk, chopped
> 3 tablespoons chopped almonds
> ½ green apple, chopped
> 1 scallion, chopped
> 2 tablespoons homemade mayonnaise
> Pinch of cayenne
> Salt to taste
> 1 small head green leaf lettuce, washed and dried

1. Mix all the ingredients (except for the lettuce).
2. Serve over a bed of greens.

■ ■ ■ SALMON CAKES WITH ASPARAGUS

These salmon cakes are a fabulous way to get your omega-3 fatty acids and still eat like a gourmet. They certainly are delicious.

SERVES 2

SALMON CAKES

> 6 ounces raw salmon, cut into small cubes
> 1 egg
> ⅓ cup ground walnuts (blended in a food processor)
> ½ cup chopped fresh Italian parsley
> ¼ teaspoon salt
> Pinch of cayenne

CAPER SAUCE

    3 tablespoons homemade mayonnaise

    1 teaspoon capers

    1 tablespoon lemon juice

    Salt to taste

    2 tablespoons chopped fresh parsley

    2 tablespoons chopped fresh dill

    ½ pound asparagus

    1 tablespoon lemon juice

    1 teaspoon olive oil

    Salt to taste

1. Mix the salmon cake ingredients and refrigerate for 1 hour.
2. Mix the caper sauce in a small bowl.
3. Chop the woody ends off the asparagus, and bring 2 inches of water to boil in a deep skillet.
4. Add the asparagus, turn down to simmer for 5 minutes.
5. Form 2 cakes with the salmon mixture.
6. Broil the cakes in a greased baking dish for 5 to 7 minutes on each side.
7. Drain the asparagus, drizzle with lemon juice and olive oil, and add a pinch of salt.
8. Serve the cakes with the caper sauce.

■ ■ ■ SCRAMBLED TOFU

Tofu for breakfast? I bet you'll like this even better than scrambled eggs!

SERVES 2

    2 tablespoons ghee (clarified butter)

    ½ onion, chopped

    1 bunch chard, washed and chopped

    ½ red bell pepper, chopped

2 garlic cloves, minced

½ cake tofu, crumbled

2 tablespoons tamari

1 teaspoon paprika

¼ cup chopped macadamia nuts

2 tablespoons chopped basil

1. In a medium skillet add the ghee and heat until nice and hot.
2. Add the onion, stir, add 2 tablespoons water, cover, turn down to medium heat, and sauté for 5 minutes.
3. Fill a large saucepan one-quater full with water, bring to a boil, add the chard, and simmer for 5 minutes.
4. To the skillet add the bell pepper and garlic, and sauté 5 more minutes.
5. Add the tofu, tamari, paprika, and basil, and cook uncovered, for 5 to 10 minutes.
6. Drain the chard and add to the skillet.
7. Sauté for 2 more minutes, then serve garnished with macadamia nuts.

■ ■ ■ ASPARAGUS SOUP AND DEVILED EGGS

Deviled eggs add a zing to creamy and delectable asparagus soup.

SERVES 2

SOUP

3 cups chicken broth

1 bunch asparagus, chopped

¼ teaspoon paprika

Pinch of cinnamon

Salt and pepper to taste

DEVILED EGGS

    2 eggs

    1 teaspoon homemade mayonnaise (see recipe on page 284)

    ¼ teaspoon mustard

    ¼ teaspoon salt

    Pinch of paprika

    Salt and pepper to taste

1. Bring the chicken broth to a boil and add the asparagus; turn down to simmer.
2. Add the paprika and cinnamon and simmer for 15 minutes, purée in food processor, and add salt and pepper.
3. Place the eggs in a saucepan, cover with cold water, bring to a boil, turn down to simmer, and simmer for 15 minutes.
4. Drain, cool the eggs in cold water, and remove the shells.
5. Slice the eggs in half lengthwise, gently remove the yolks, and place in a small bowl with the mayonnaise, mustard, and salt. Blend with a fork. Using a small spoon, fill the egg whites with the yolk mixture.

■ ■ ■ CHICKEN TARRAGON

Cooking the chicken and herbs for a long time imparts a rich flavor.

SERVES 2

    1 onion, chopped

    2 tablespoons ghee (clarified butter)

    3 shiitake mushrooms, stems removed, sliced

    3 boneless, skinless chicken breasts (one is for Mesclun and Chicken Salad
        tomorrow, page 239)

    5 cups chicken broth

    ¼ cup chopped fresh tarragon

    1 tablespoon chopped fresh thyme

    2 bunches spinach, well washed

    ¼ cup chopped cashews

1. Sauté the onion in ghee in a large skillet on medium heat for 5 minutes.
2. Add the shiitakes and sauté for 3 minutes more.
3. Add the chicken breasts and brown each side.
4. Add the broth and herbs, cover, and simmer for about 2 hours, making sure that the chicken is covered with liquid, adding broth as necessary.
5. Steam the spinach in a veggie steamer, and divide between two plates.
6. Top with the chicken breasts, plenty of broth, and cashews.

■ ■ ■ ROASTED PEPPER TOASTS

This is a Sunday brunch treat for bread lovers.

SERVES 2

> 1 red bell pepper
> ¼ cup pine nuts
> 1 garlic clove
> 2 tablespoons extra virgin olive oil
> 1 teaspoon chopped fresh rosemary
> 2 tablespoons cream cheese
> 2 slices "Manna from Heaven" bread

1. Roast the bell pepper on an open flame on the stovetop or broil in the oven, then place in a brown paper bag.
2. When cool, peel the skin off the pepper, cut in half, remove the seeds and stem, and place it in a food processor with the pine nuts, garlic, olive oil, and rosemary.
3. Toast the Manna bread, spread on the cream cheese, and top with pepper spread.

■ ■ ■ MESCLUN AND CHICKEN SALAD

Adding the essence from last night's Chicken Tarragon (page 237) gives this salad its punch.

SERVES 2

>   3 handfuls mesclun salad mix
>   ½ cup snow peas
>   ¼ cup chopped walnuts
>   Leftover Chicken Tarragon, cut into bite-sized pieces
>   2 tablespoons grated Parmesan

TARRAGON DRESSING

>   3 tablespoons tarragon essence (broth from Chicken Tarragon)
>   2 tablespoons extra virgin olive oil
>   1 tablespoon fresh lemon juice
>   1 tablespoon chopped fresh tarragon
>   Salt to taste

1. To a large salad bowl add the lettuce, snow peas, walnuts, chicken, and Parmesan.
2. Add the dressing, toss, and serve.

■ ■ ■ ROASTED CORNISH GAME HENS

Cornish game hens are quite delectable, but if you can't find them, you can substitute a roasting chicken.

SERVES 2

>   2 Cornish game hens
>   2 lemon wedges
>   2 sprigs fresh rosemary

2 sprigs fresh thyme

12 sprigs Italian parsley

2 sprigs fresh sage

3 medium leeks, chopped

4 garlic cloves, peeled

3 stalks celery, cut into 2-inch chunks

2 turnips, quartered

2 tablespoons butter

¼ teaspoon salt

Pinch of black pepper

1. Preheat the oven to 425°F.
2. Stuff each hen with 1 lemon wedge and a small bundle of rosemary, thyme, parsley, and sage.
3. Place the hens in a roasting pan and arrange the leeks, garlic, celery, and turnips around them.
4. Put several dots of butter on top of each hen, sprinkle with salt and pepper, and place in the oven.
5. Turn the oven down to 350°F and bake for 1 hour, or until juices run clear.

■ ■ ■ ARUGULA SALAD

Arugula is also known as rocket. This spicy salad is sure to send your taste buds into orbit.

SERVES 2

DRESSING

½ cup extra virgin olive oil

2 tablespoons balsamic vinegar

½ teaspoon Dijon mustard

Salt to taste

Stevia powder (or other sugar substitute) to taste

    1 bunch arugula, washed and dried
    ¼ cup slivered almonds
    ¼ cup Parmesan (shaved with a carrot peeler)

1. Mix the dressing in a small bowl with a fork.
2. Combine the arugula, almonds, and Parmesan in a salad bowl, toss with dressing, and enjoy.

■ ■ ■ SMOOTHIE WITH HAZELNUTS

A great variation on a familiar theme

SERVES 2

    2 scoops whey protein powder
    1 teaspoon flax oil
    ¼ cup hazelnuts, skinless
    ½ cup strawberries, washed, with tops removed
    16 ounces pure water
    Pinch of cinnamon

Mix all the ingredients in a blender.

■ ■ ■ ROMAINE SALAD À LA RON

This is a really great main course salad. The combination of macadamia nuts, avocado, and Jarlsberg cheese (my favorite) makes this salad something really special.

SERVES 2

    1 head romaine lettuce, washed and dried
    1 hard-boiled egg, chopped

1 ripe avocado, peeled, pitted, and chopped

¼ cup chopped macadamia nuts

2 tablespoons grated Jarlsberg

DRESSING

⅔ cup walnut oil

2 tablespoons fresh lemon juice

1 garlic clove

¼ cup chopped fresh basil

Salt and pepper to taste

1. Mix the dressing ingredients in a blender.
2. Add all the other ingredients to a salad bowl, add the dressing, toss, and serve.

■ ■ ■ BROILED SCALLOPS

Decadent yet healthy, this is one to serve at your next dinner party.

SERVES 2

1 pound scallops

6 thinly sliced baby bok choy

¼ cup chopped fresh Italian parsley

3 tablespoons ghee (clarified butter), melted

2 tablespoons chopped hazelnuts

2 lime wedges

¼ teaspoon salt

1. Rinse the scallops and pat dry.
2. Steam the bok choy for 7 minutes.
3. Preheat the oven to broil.
4. Toss the scallops with the parsley and ghee in a small glass baking dish.
5. Broil for 5 to 10 minutes, depending on the size of the scallops.

6. Arrange the bok choy on plates, spoon the scallop mixture over, top with hazelnuts, and serve with lime wedges.
7. Salt to taste.

■ ■ ■ POACHED EGGS OVER GREENS WITH ROASTED RED PEPPER SAUCE

No, not green eggs and ham, but eggs and greens smothered in an irresistible sauce.

SERVES 2

SAUCE

  1 red bell pepper
  1 garlic clove
  ¼ cup extra virgin olive oil
  ¼ cup macadamia nuts
  ¼ cup chopped fresh basil
  Salt to taste

  2 eggs
  2 bunches green chard, washed and chopped

1. Roast the bell pepper (see page 238).
2. Let cool in a paper bag, remove the skin, cut in half, and remove the seeds and stem.
3. Combine the bell pepper, garlic, olive oil, macadamia nuts, basil, and salt in a food processor.
4. Fill a large saucepan one-third full of water and bring to a boil, add the chard to the saucepan, reduce the heat, and simmer for 5 minutes.
5. Poach the eggs (see page 215).
6. Drain the chard and arrange on plates, top with the eggs.
7. Drench with sauce and serve.

■ ■ ■ POACHED SALMON SALAD

Salmon and dill go so well together. They are especially nice in this fresh salad, with naturally sweet and crunchy pecans and creamy chèvre.

SERVES 2

> 2 3-ounce salmon fillets
> 4 cups baby romaine lettuce, washed and dried
> 1 endive, thinly sliced
> 2 tablespoons chèvre
> ¼ cup pecans

DILL DRESSING

> ½ cup avocado oil
> ¼ cup yogurt
> 3 tablespoons fresh lemon juice
> ¼ cup chopped fresh dill
> Salt to taste

1. Rinse the fillets and pat dry.
2. Place the fish in a large skillet, add enough boiling water, to cover the fish, and simmer for 10 minutes.
3. Divide the salad greens and endive between two plates and dot each with chèvre.
4. Roast the pecans in a cast-iron skillet until they start to make a sizzling sound, then cool on a plate.
5. Mix the dressing in a blender.
6. Top each salad with a salmon fillet and pecans, pour the dressing over, and serve.

▪ ▪ ▪ BAKED HALIBUT IN PESTO SAUCE

Pesto adds flavor and texture to mild, meaty halibut.

SERVES 2

PESTO

>2 cups fresh basil leaves
>
>½ cup extra virgin olive oil
>
>¼ cup walnuts
>
>2 tablespoons grated Parmesan
>
>3 garlic cloves

>2 3-ounce halibut fillets

>½ pound Brussels sprouts
>
>3 tablespoons fresh lemon juice
>
>1 teaspoon lemon zest
>
>2 tablespoons chopped fresh parsley
>
>Salt and black pepper

1. Preheat the oven to 400°F.
2. Mix the pesto in a blender. (Save 2 tablespoons for tomorrow's breakfast, page 246.)
3. Rinse the fish and pat dry.
4. Place a large piece of aluminum foil in the bottom of a glass baking dish.
5. Spoon a layer of pesto on the foil, place the fillets on the foil, and spoon more pesto on top.
6. Fold the foil around the fish to make a little package.
7. Bake for 20 minutes, or until the fish is opaque throughout.
8. Fill a large saucepan half full with water, bring to a boil, add the Brussels sprouts, and reduce to a simmer for 7 to 10 minutes.
9. Drain the Brussels sprouts; add lemon juice, lemon zest, parsley, and salt and pepper.

■ ■ ■ "MANNA FROM HEAVEN" BREAD WITH PESTO AND TURKEY SAUSAGE

This is a hearty and easy-to-prepare breakfast.

SERVES 2

Pesto, left over from last night's Baked Halibut (page 245)

2 turkey sausage patties

2 pieces "Manna from Heaven" bread, toasted

1. Preheat the oven to broil.
2. Broil the sausage patties for 5 minutes on each side, or until done.
3. Spread the toast with pesto.
4. Top with sausage and serve.

■ ■ ■ COTTAGE CHEESE AND SAUTÉED KALE

Spicy cayenne and kale dress up simple cottage cheese.

SERVES 2

1 bunch kale, washed and chopped

1 garlic clove, minced

Extra virgin olive oil

Salt to taste

Pinch or two of cayenne

1 cup low-fat cottage cheese

1. Sauté the kale and garlic in the olive oil in a heavy skillet.
2. Split between two plates; add salt and cayenne.
3. Top with half a cup of cottage cheese per plate, and serve.

■ ■ ■ CURRIED CHICKEN

Need a little comfort food? This warming dish is just the thing!

SERVES 2

> 1 onion, chopped
> 3 tablespoons ghee (clarified butter)
> 2 boneless, skinless chicken breasts
> 2 tablespoons curry powder
> 3 garlic cloves, minced
> 1 can low-fat coconut milk
> 2 bunches spinach, well washed
> Stevia powder to taste

1. Sauté the onion in the ghee in a large skillet for 5 minutes.
2. Rinse the chicken breasts and slice diagonally into strips.
3. Add the curry powder, garlic, and 3 tablespoons water to the skillet, and simmer for 3 more minutes.
4. Add the chicken breasts, stir, cover, and simmer for 5 minutes, then add the coconut milk and simmer for 20 to 30 more minutes, making sure that the chicken is covered with liquid.
5. Steam the spinach.
6. Sweeten the curry with Stevia (or Spenda) to taste.
7. Serve the curry over a bed of spinach.

■ ■ ■ TOFU AND BROCCOLI WITH LEMONY ALMOND SAUCE

Here's another tasty tofu dish that's simple to make.

SERVES 2

> ½ cake tofu
> 1 tablespoon olive oil

    1 tablespoon tamari

    2 tablespoons chopped almonds

SAUCE

    3 tablespoons chopped almonds

    1 tablespoon tamari

    1 garlic clove, minced

    2 to 3 tablespoons fresh lemon juice

    2 tablespoons extra virgin olive oil

    2 cups broccoli florets

1. Preheat the oven to 400°F.
2. Cut the tofu into small cubes.
3. Toss the tofu with the olive oil and tamari, place in a glass baking dish, and bake for about 30 minutes.
4. Mix the sauce in a blender.
5. Steam the broccoli.
6. Toss the tofu and broccoli with sauce, split between two plates, top with chopped almonds, and serve.

■ ■ ■ GRILLED MAHIMAHI

Mahimahi always tastes delicious to me, but with this sauce it is absolutely mouthwatering!

SERVES 2

    2 4-ounce mahimahi fillets

    2 tablespoons extra virgin olive oil

    ¼ teaspoon salt

    ¼ teaspoon pepper

SAUCE

  ¼ cup ghee (clarified butter), melted

  3 tablespoons fresh lemon juice

  2 garlic cloves

  2 scallions, chopped

  Pinch of cayenne

1. Preheat grill to medium heat.
2. Rub the mahimahi fillets with extra virgin oil. Sprinkle with salt and pepper.
3. Mix the sauce ingredients in a small bowl.
4. Grill mahimahi fillets for 5 minutes on each side, or until opaque throughout.
5. Remove from heat. Place each fillet on a serving plate. Pour sauce over fillets and serve with Grilled Veggies (see below).

■ ■ ■ GRILLED VEGGIES

Great with Grilled Mahimahi (see above).

SERVES 2

  2 eggplant, sliced into rounds

  1 onion, cut in quarters

  2 zucchini, sliced in rounds

  2 red bell peppers, cut in quarters

BASIL VINAIGRETTE

  1 cup olive oil

  ½ cup chopped fresh basil

  3 tablespoons balsamic vinegar

  Pinch of cayenne

  Salt to taste

  Stevia powder or (Splenda) to taste

1. Marinade the veggies in the basil vinaigrette for 1 hour.
2. Preheat oven to 400°F.
3. Place the veggies in a glass baking dish, cover with aluminum foil, and bake until tender, approximately 20 minutes.
4. Transfer the veggies to a grill and grill for 5 to 10 minutes on each side, and save some for tomorrow's lunch (Roasted Veggie Wrap, below).

▪ ▪ ▪ ROASTED VEGGIE WRAP

Encore!

SERVES 2

2 tortillas (use only low-carb La Tortilla Factory tortillas)
2 tablespoons low fat cream cheese
Veggies left over from last night's Grilled Veggies (page 249)
¼ cup chopped fresh basil

1. Lay the tortillas on a large cutting board.
2. Spread each with a thin layer of cream cheese.
3. Arrange the veggies in a thick strip two-thirds toward the bottom of each tortilla.
4. Place the basil leaves in a row above the veggies.
5. Roll the tortillas, slice into rounds, and serve.

▪ ▪ ▪ TRISH'S TUNA

This mouthwatering, easy-to-prepare recipe was created by Jena's mother. For the best results, marinate the tuna overnight.

SERVES 2

2 4-ounce tuna steaks

TUNA MARINADE

½ cup chopped fresh rosemary

12 garlic cloves, chopped

1½ cups extra virgin olive oil

Pinch of salt

Dash of black pepper

2 cups cauliflower florets

2 tablespoons fresh lemon juice

1 tablespoon capers

2 tablespoons extra virgin olive oil

3 tablespoons chopped macadamia nuts

Salt and pepper to taste

1. Marinate the tuna overnight in a glass baking dish or Ziploc bag.
2. Preheat the grill.
3. Steam the cauliflower.
4. Grill the tuna for 5 minutes each side.
5. Toss the cauliflower with lemon juice, capers, olive oil, macadamia nuts, and salt and pepper, and serve.

■ ■ ■ TOASTED "MANNA FROM HEAVEN" BREAD WITH AVOCADO, SMOKED SALMON, DILL, AND POACHED EGGS

Another version of eggs and toast with delicious complements.

SERVES 2

2 eggs

2 pieces smoked salmon

2 slices "Manna from Heaven" bread, toasted

1 ripe avocado, sliced
2 tablespoons chopped fresh dill
Salt and pepper

1. Poach the eggs (see Eggs "Benefit," page 215).
2. Place a piece of salmon on top of each slice of toasted Manna bread.
3. Place sliced avocado on top of the salmon, top the avocado with the eggs, and sprinkle with dill, salt, and pepper.

■ ■ ■ FISH CHOWDER

Leeks are the secret ingredient in this flavorful soup.

SERVES 2

3 leeks, chopped
2 tablespoons extra virgin olive oil
3 cups chicken broth
4 celery stalks, chopped
2 cups cauliflower florets
2 garlic cloves, chopped
1 tablespoon chopped fresh thyme
2 tablespoons chopped fresh basil
1 6-ounce cod fillet, cut into small pieces
Salt to taste
Pinch of cayenne
Chopped fresh parsley

1. Sauté the leeks in the olive oil for 5 minutes.
2. Add ¼ cup of the chicken broth, celery, cauliflower, garlic, and herbs; cover and cook for 10 minutes.
3. Add the cod and the rest of the chicken broth, and simmer for 30 minutes.
4. Add salt and cayenne, and serve garnished with parsley.

■ ■ ■ TOFU PORTOBELLO CASSEROLE

The meaty texture of the portobellos, the sweetness of the tomatoes, and the delicate flavor and aroma of fresh basil blend very nicely.

SERVES 2

> 1 cake tofu
>
> 5 portobellos mushrooms, 3 thinly sliced and 2 kept whole for tomorrow's lunch (Mesclun Mix Salad, page 254)
>
> 1 cup cherry tomatoes
>
> 1 cup chopped fresh basil
>
> 3 tablespoons tamari (soy sauce sold in health food stores.)
>
> Extra virgin olive oil
>
> Stevia powder to taste
>
> 1 bunch chard, washed, stems removed, and chopped

1. Preheat the oven to 400°F.
2. Cut the tofu into large triangles.
3. In an oiled glass baking dish, mix the sliced portobellos and the rest of the ingredients well.
4. Cover the dish with aluminum foil and bake for 30 minutes, remove foil and bake for 10 more minutes.
5. Steam the chard for 5 minutes.
6. Serve the tofu casserole over a bed of chard.

■ ■ ■ MESCLUN MIX SALAD

Here's another tasty salad with great textures.

SERVES 2

BASIL VINAIGRETTE (SEE RECIPE ON PAGE 230)

> 4 cups mesclun salad mix
>
> 2 whole portobello mushroom caps, sliced, from last night's Tofu Portobello Casserole (page 253)
>
> 4 tablespoons chèvre
>
> 1 small endive, sliced
>
> ¼ cup chopped fresh basil
>
> ¼ cup walnuts, roughly chopped

1. Blend the salad dressing.
2. Mix all the ingredients in a salad bowl, pour the dressing over, toss, and serve.

■ ■ ■ GRILLED BEEF FILLETS WITH BELL PEPPERS AND MASHED RUTABAGAS

This dinner is simple to prepare, full of flavor, and very satisfying.

SERVES 2

> 3 4-ounce tenderloin fillets (save one for Steak and Soft-Boiled Eggs tomorrow, page 255)
>
> 1 green bell pepper, cut in quarters
>
> 1 red bell pepper, cut in quarters
>
> 3 medium rutabagas, peeled and cut into chunks
>
> 1 fennel root, cut in half
>
> 1 tablespoon butter

1 tablespoon of cream
Salt to taste
Pinch of cayenne

1. Rub the fillets with olive oil and sprinkle with salt and pepper.
2. Fill a large sauce pan one-half full with water, bring to a boil, and add rutabagas and fennel. Turn down to simmer for 15 to 20 minutes or until you can easily slide a fork into them.
3. Preheat the grill.
4. Fill a medium sauce pan one-half full with water. Bring to a boil. Add peppers and simmer for 5 minutes. Remove peppers.
5. Drain rutabagas and fennel, add to the food processor, and blend with butter, salt, cayenne, and cream.
6. Grill green peppers for 5 minutes on each side. Set aside on platter.
7. Grill two fillets for 8 to 10 minutes on each side, and one for 5 minutes on each side. (This one is for tomorrow's breakfast, Steak and Soft-Boiled Eggs, below.) Serve with vegetables.

■ ■ ■ STEAK AND SOFT-BOILED EGGS

What's for breakfast? That's right, here's the beef!

SERVES 2

Leftover fillet from Grilled Beef Fillets with Bell Peppers and Mashed Rutabagas
(see above)
2 eggs
Salt and pepper to taste

1. Cut the extra steak into strips and heat in a skillet on both sides.
2. Soft-boil the eggs, and serve.

■ ■ ■ BERRY GOOD SALAD

The hint of sweetness that blueberries add to this salad is refreshing.

SERVES 2

DIJON VINAIGRETTE (SEE RECIPE ON PAGE 216)

- 1 head romaine lettuce, washed and dried
- ¼ cup grated Jarlsberg
- ¼ cup sprouts
- 1 ripe avocado, sliced
- ¼ cup blueberries
- ¼ cup cashews

Toss all the salad ingredients together, pour the vinaigrette over, and serve.

■ ■ ■ TURKEY BURGER, MUSTARD GREENS, FETA, AND BLACK PEPPER

A hearty, healthy version of the all-American burger.

SERVES 2

- ½ pound ground turkey
- 1 egg white
- 3 tablespoons ground almonds (blended in a food processor)
- Salt and pepper
- Pinch of cayenne
- 1 bunch mustard greens, washed and chopped
- 2 tablespoons crumbled sheep's feta
- Black pepper to taste

1. Preheat the grill.
2. Mix the turkey, egg white, almonds, salt, pepper, and cayenne.
3. Make into patties.
4. Fill a large saucepan one-third full of water and bring to a boil.
5. Add the mustard greens to the pan, reduce to simmer, and simmer for 10 minutes.
6. Grill the burgers for 10 to 15 minutes on each side, or until done.
7. Top each patty with feta for the last few minutes of grilling.
8. Drain the mustard greens, divide between two plates, top with the burgers and black pepper, and serve.

■ ■ ■ POACHED EGG ON "MANNA FROM HEAVEN" BREAD WITH PESTO

Pesto adds a little spice to poached eggs.

SERVES 2

> 2 poached eggs (see Eggs "Benefit," page 215)
> 2 slices "Manna from Heaven" bread, toasted

PESTO (SEE BAKED HALIBUT IN PESTO SAUCE, PAGE 245)

Spoon the pesto sauce over the poached eggs on toast.

■ ■ ■ TOFU WRAP

Wrap it up and take it to lunch!

SERVES 2

> ½ cake tofu
> 2 tablespoons extra virgin olive oil
> 1 tablespoon tamari

AVOCADO SPREAD

1 ripe avocado

1 garlic clove

1 teaspoon fresh lemon juice

¼ cup chopped fresh cilantro

Dash of cayenne

1 cup grated carrots

1 cup sunflower sprouts

2 low-carb La Tortilla Factory tortillas

1. Preheat the oven to 400°F.
2. Cut the tofu into cubes, toss with olive oil and tamari, and bake for 20 minutes.
3. Blend the avocado spread in a food processor.
4. Spread each tortilla with a layer of avocado spread.
5. Place the tofu in a line horizontally about two-thirds toward the bottom of each tortilla.
6. Place a line of carrots and sprouts above the tofu.
7. Roll the tortillas and serve.

■ ■ ■ DIJON SALMON SERVED WITH STEAMED GREEN BEANS

King or Coho salmon taste the best. Keep it wild, not farm raised!

SERVES 2 WITH LEFTOVERS (SAVE TO USE IN BABY ROMAINE SALAD, PAGE 260, TOMORROW).

1 10-ounce salmon fillet

SAUCE

2 tablespoons Dijon mustard

1 tablespoon tamari

1 cup raspberries

2 tablespoons water

2 handfuls green beans, ends snipped

1 tablespoon avocado oil

1 tablespoon fresh lemon juice

2 tablespoons chopped fresh parsley

Salt to taste

1. Rinse the fish, pat dry, and place in a glass baking dish, skin side up.
2. Pour the sauce over the salmon, and marinate in the refrigerator for 1 hour.
3. Preheat the oven to 400°F.
4. Bake the salmon, covered with aluminum foil, for 10 minutes, then turn skin side down and bake for approximately 10 more minutes depending on the thickness of the fish.
5. Fill a large saucepan one-half full with water and bring to a boil, add the green beans, reduce to a simmer for 7 minutes.
6. Drain the beans and toss with avocado oil, lemon juice, parsley, and salt.

■ ■ ■ TURKEY SAUSAGE WITH POACHED EGGS

Get up and go!

SERVES 2

2 turkey sausages

2 poached eggs (see Eggs "Benefit," page 215)

Salt to taste

Pinch of cayenne

1. Broil the sausages for 5 minutes on each side, blot excess oil with paper towels, and place on plates.
2. Top with poached eggs, sprinkle with salt and cayenne, and serve.

■ ■ ■ BABY ROMAINE SALAD

Leftover salmon from Dijon Salmon with Steamed Green Beans is the
secret touch in this delectable salad.

SERVES 2

DRESSING

- ¼ cup leftover salmon sauce
- 2 tablespoons extra virgin olive oil
- 1 tablespoon fresh lemon juice
- Dash of cider vinegar
- Salt to taste
- Pinch of cayenne

- 3 cups baby romaine lettuce, washed and dried
- 4 ounces leftover salmon broken into bite-sized pieces (see Dijon Salmon Served with
  Steamed Green Beans, page 258)
- ¼ cup chopped walnuts
- ½ cup chopped fresh basil
- 1 small head radicchio

1. Mix the dressing in a small bowl with a fork.
2. Add all the other ingredients to a salad bowl, add the dressing, toss,
   and serve.

■ ■ ■ GRILLED CHICKEN WITH CILANTRO PESTO AND STEAMED KALE

The cilantro and lime juice in this dish give it a bit of Southwest flavor.

SERVES 2

CILANTRO PESTO

    1 bunch cilantro, washed and chopped (save a few sprigs for garnish)
    2 to 3 garlic cloves
    ¼ cup extra virgin olive oil
    1 tablespoon chèvre
    1 to 2 teaspoons lime juice
    2 boneless, skinless chicken breasts
    Extra virgin olive oil
    Salt and pepper
    1 bunch kale, washed and chopped

1. Mix the pesto in a food processor.
2. Preheat the grill.
3. Wash the chicken breasts, pat dry, rub with olive oil, and sprinkle with salt and pepper.
4. Grill the chicken on medium heat for about 10 minutes each side. Cut into the middle of breasts to test for doneness. The color should be white and juices should run clear.
5. Steam the kale.
6. Slice the chicken on the diagonal and spoon a generous amount of pesto on top.
7. Garnish with chopped cilantro.

■ ■ ■ BROCCOLI SOUP

This is a great way to get kids to eat broccoli and enjoy it yourself.

SERVES 2

    3 tablespoons ghee (clarified butter)
    1 red onion, chopped
    2 garlic cloves
    4 cup chicken broth
    4 cups chopped broccoli, flowers and tender stems

1 cake silken tofu, cut into chunks
½ cup chopped almonds
1 teaspoon salt
½ teaspoon paprika
Pinch of cayenne

1. In a large soup pot, melt ghee, add the onions, and sauté for 5 minutes.
2. Add the garlic and chicken broth and bring to a boil.
3. Add broccoli and reduce to simmer for 10 minutes, then remove from heat.
4. Blend the soup in batches in a food processor, adding the tofu, almonds, salt, paprika, and cayenne to taste. Serve warm.

■ ■ ■ HALIBUT WITH LIME AND CILANTRO SERVED WITH ASPARAGUS

This sauce adds a piquant flavor to halibut.

SERVES 2

2 4-ounce halibut fillets

SAUCE

¼ cup fresh lime juice
½ cup chopped fresh cilantro
3 tablespoons extra virgin olive oil
Pinch of cayenne

1. Preheat the oven to 400°F.
2. Rinse the fish and pat dry with a paper towel.
3. Place the fish skin side up, in a glass baking dish, pour the sauce over, and bake covered for 5 minutes, then turn the fish over and bake for another 5 to 10 minutes, or until opaque throughout.

▪ ▪ ▪ GRILLED SALMON AND STEAMED CHARD

Simple but very satisfying.

SERVES 2

> 2 3-ounce salmon fillets
> 2 tablespoons extra virgin olive oil
> 2 garlic cloves, chopped
> ¼ cup fresh lemon juice
> 1 bunch chard, washed, chopped, and steamed
> 2 tablespoons chopped fresh parsley

1. Preheat the grill.
2. Rinse the fillets, pat dry, and rub with olive oil and garlic.
3. Grill the salmon for 5 minutes each side.
4. Make a bed of chard on each plate, top with the salmon, pour lemon juice over, and sprinkle with parsley.

▪ ▪ ▪ PIZZA WITH PESTO SAUCE

Pizza without the guilt!

SERVES 2

CRUST

> 1 cup finely chopped walnuts (in a food processor)
> ½ cup coarsely chopped walnuts
> 2 cups grated zucchini
> ¼ cup extra virgin olive oil
> ¼ teaspoon salt

Pesto (see Baked Halibut in Pesto Sauce, on page 245)

TOPPING

>½ cup canned-in-water artichoke hearts, chopped
>
>2 garlic cloves, chopped
>
>½ cup crumbled sheep's feta
>
>½ cup chopped fresh basil leaves

1. Preheat the oven to 375°F.
2. Mix the crust ingredients and press onto an oiled baking sheet.
3. Bake the crust for 15 to 20 minutes, or until it begins to brown.
4. Remove from the oven and spread a thick layer of pesto sauce on the crust.
5. Top with the artichoke hearts, garlic, feta, and basil.
6. Place in the oven for several more minutes, remove, slice, and serve.

■ ■ ■ COUNTRY FRENCH SOUP

This is a low-carb version of everybody's favorite French soup.

SERVES 2 WITH LEFTOVERS

>4 leeks well washed and chopped, greens and all
>
>2 tablespoons olive oil
>
>3 celery stalks, chopped
>
>3 carrots, sliced into rounds
>
>1½ cups fresh green beans, cut into thirds
>
>1 cup canned navy beans, rinsed
>
>4 cups canned or fresh chicken broth
>
>1 teaspoon salt
>
>¼ teaspoon pepper
>
>⅛ cup fresh grated Parmesan

FRENCH PESTO, OR PISTOU

>1 cup basil
>
>¼ cup olive oil
>
>2 cloves garlic

1. Mix the pesto ingredients in a food processor.
2. Saute the leeks in the olive oil and 3 teaspoons broth; when soft, add the celery, carrots, and ½ cup chicken broth, and simmer for 5 minutes.
3. Add the remaining broth, return to a simmer, add the green beans, and simmer for 3 minutes.
4. Add the navy beans and simmer for 5 more minutes. Add salt and pepper.
5. Serve immediately, each bowl topped with 1 tablespoon pesto and 1 teaspoon Parmesan.

■ ■ ■ BLACK COD

The colors and flavors in this easy-to-prepare dish are vibrant.

SERVES 2

2 6-ounce black cod fillets (one is for tomorrow's Sea and Green Salad, page 266)

2 bunches spinach, well washed and blanched

1 cup cherry tomatoes

½ cup black olives, pitted and chopped

2 tablespoons chopped fresh parsley

1 garlic clove, chopped

3 tablespoons fresh lemon juice

2 tablespoons olive oil

¼ cup chopped fresh basil

1. Rinse the cod fillets and pat dry.
2. Preheat the oven to 400°F.
3. Put the blanched spinach in a glass baking dish, top with the fish, and surround with the cherry tomatoes, olives, and garlic.
4. Pour the lemon juice and olive oil on the fish and veggies, and top with basil and parsley.
5. Bake for 5 minutes, covered with aluminum foil, remove the foil; and bake for 5 to 10 more minutes, or until opaque throughout.

6. Save one piece of fish for tomorrow's lunch (Sea and Green Salad, below).

■ ■ ■ SOFT-BOILED EGGS AND "MANNA FROM HEAVEN" BREAD WITH SAUSAGE SAUCE

Here's a new meaty sauce to try.

SERVES 2

SAUSAGE SAUCE

    1 turkey sausage patty, broiled
    1 tablespoon melted ghee (clarified butter)
    ¼ cup cream
    Salt to taste
    ¼ teaspoon paprika

    2 pieces "Manna from Heaven" bread, toasted
    2 soft-boiled eggs (see Eggs "Benefit," page 215)

1. Mix the sausage sauce in a blender, adding a little water for a thinner sauce.
2. Place the eggs on top of the toast, cut just the eggs in half, cover with the sauce, and serve.

■ ■ ■ SEA AND GREEN SALAD

Pine nuts and sun-dried tomatoes add an Italian flavor to this quick lunch.

SERVES 2

BALSAMIC VINAIGRETTE (SEE RECIPE ON PAGE 219)

>   1 head romaine lettuce, washed and dried
>
>   3 tablespoons chèvre
>
>   ¼ cup chopped sun-dried tomatoes, packed in olive oil
>
>   Leftover black cod, broken into bite-sized pieces (see Black Cod, page 265)
>
>   ½ cup pine nuts, toasted
>
>   2 tablespoons chopped fresh basil

1. Blend the vinaigrette.
2. Combine all the rest of the ingredients in a large salad bowl, pour the dressing over, toss well, and serve.

■ ■ ■ SHEPHERD'S PIE

You can substitute ground beef if you prefer; either way this is a very hearty, rich, savory meal.

SERVES 2 WITH LEFTOVERS

>   1 head cauliflower, cut into florets
>
>   1 tablespoon olive oil
>
>   1 bunch chard, washed and chopped
>
>   1 large chopped onion
>
>   3 chopped carrots
>
>   1 cup beef stock
>
>   3 to 4 garlic cloves, chopped
>
>   3 tablespoons chopped fresh rosemary
>
>   ¼ cup chopped fresh Italian parsley
>
>   1 tablespoon chopped fresh thyme
>
>   ¾ pound ground lamb
>
>   1 tablespoon xanthan gum
>
>   1 tablespoon butter
>
>   Salt to taste
>
>   Black pepper, coarsely ground to taste

1. Bring a medium saucepan one-half full with water to a boil, turn down to simmer, add the cauliflower, and simmer for 10 minutes.
2. To a large, deep skillet add the olive oil, heat, and add the onion.
3. Sauté the onion, adding 2 tablespoons of the beef broth, garlic, and herbs.
4. When the onion is translucent, add the carrots and chard, and simmer for 5 more minutes.
5. Add the lamb and sauté until browned.
6. Add the remaining beef broth, return to simmer, and stir in the xanthan gum to thicken.
7. Reduce the heat to low, cover, and simmer, for 5 minutes.
8. Preheat the oven to 425°F.
9. Blend the cauliflower in a food processor with butter, salt, and pepper.
10. Add the lamb mixture to a large glass pie plate and top with cauliflower.
11. Dot the cauliflower with butter and bake, uncovered, for about 7 minutes, or until it begins to brown a bit.

■ ■ ■ SMOKED SALMON WITH CREAM CHEESE ON "MANNA FROM HEAVEN" BREAD

You can make this breakfast in a flash.

SERVES 2

2 tablespoons low-fat cream cheese
2 slices "Manna bread from Heaven"; toasted
6 ounces smoked salmon

Spread the cream cheese on the toast, top with the salmon, and serve.

■ ■ ■ CHICKEN WRAP

Here's a yummy lunch wrap.

SERVES 2

  1 boneless, skinless chicken breast
  1 tablespoon extra virgin olive oil
  Salt and pepper
  2 low-carb La Tortilla Factory tortillas
  Pesto (see Baked Halibut in Pesto Sauce, page 245)
  ¼ cup chopped sun-dried tomatoes
  3 tablespoons chèvre

1. Preheat the grill.
2. Rub the chicken with olive oil, salt, and pepper.
3. Grill the breasts for 10 minutes each side, or until done.
4. Spread the tortillas with pesto.
5. Slice the chicken, arrange in a row two-thirds toward the bottom of each tortilla. Add the tomatoes above the chicken, crumble the chèvre on top, roll the tortillas, slice into rounds, and serve.

■ ■ ■ LASAGNA

Substitute heavy, starchy lasagna noodles with thinly sliced zucchini and summer squash.

SERVES 2

  3 large zucchini
  3 large summer squash
  3 tablespoons extra virgin olive oil

FILLING

¼ cup grated Parmesan

2 cups low-fat ricotta

1 egg

½ cup chopped fresh Italian parsley

2 bunches spinach, well washed and steamed

½ cup chopped walnuts

Basil pesto (double the recipe from Baked Halibut in Pesto Sauce, page 245)

1. Preheat the oven to 400°F.
2. Slice the zucchini and squash lengthwise, toss in olive oil, and roast on greased baking sheets for about 15 minutes, remove the veggies, and reduce the heat to 350°F.
3. Mix the filling ingredients.
4. Place one layer of roasted vegetables in the bottom of a 9 × 12-inch glass baking dish.
5. Spread a thin layer of pesto on top of the vegetables, and a layer of filling on top of the pesto vegetables, about 1 inch thick.
6. Create another layer of vegetables and another layer of filling.
7. Top with a final layer of vegetables and a layer of pesto. Sprinkle with Parmesan, and bake, covered, for 40 minutes.

■ ■ ■ BERRIES AND YOGURT

Crunchy macadamia nuts and cinnamon add a new flair to a simple breakfast.

SERVES 2

2 cups yogurt

⅓ cup blueberries

1 teaspoon lemon juice

¼ teaspoon ground cinnamon

¼ cup chopped macadamia nuts

1. Mix the yogurt, blueberries, lemon juice, and cinnamon.
2. Sprinkle macadamia nuts on top, and serve.

■ ■ ■ LENTIL SOUP

This soup is very filling and easy to put together.

SERVES 2 WITH LEFTOVERS

2 cups dried lentils

1 onion, chopped

1-inch piece of fresh ginger, peeled and chopped

4 garlic cloves, chopped

3 tablespoons extra virgin olive oil

1 quart chicken stock

1 quart water

½ cup chopped fresh parsley

1 large bunch chard, washed and chopped

¼ cup fresh lemon juice

1 teaspoon salt

¼ teaspoon black pepper

¼ teaspoon cinnamon

1. Rinse the lentils well in a large colander.
2. Sauté the onion, ginger, and garlic in olive oil.
3. Add the lentils, stock, and water, cover, bring to a boil, and reduce to simmer.
4. Simmer for 2 hours, add parsley and chard, and simmer for 20 to 30 more minutes.
5. Blend half of the soup in a food processor, return to the pot, add lemon juice, cinnamon, salt, and pepper, and serve.

■ ■ ■ TILAPIA IN ROASTED RED BELL PEPPER SAUCE WITH SNOW PEAS

This sauce adds nice color and spice to tilapia.

SERVES 2

> 1 8-ounce tilapia fillet
> 2 tablespoons walnut oil
> Salt and pepper
> Pinch of cayenne
> 2 handfuls snow peas
> 2 tablespoons chopped fresh mint
> 2 tablespoons grated Parmesan
> Extra virgin olive oil
> Roasted red pepper sauce (see recipe on page 243)

1. Preheat the oven to broil.
2. Rub the fish with the oil, sprinkle with salt and pepper, and broil for 5 minutes on each side.
3. Steam the snow peas for 5 minutes, then toss with the mint, Parmesan, salt, and olive oil.
4. Arrange the fillets on plates, lavish with red bell pepper sauce, and serve with the snow peas.

■ ■ ■ POACHED EGGS OVER TOMATO WITH PESTO

SERVES 2

> 2 eggs
> 1 tomato
> Pesto (see Baked Halibut in Pesto Sauce, page 245)

1. Poach the eggs (see Eggs "Benefit," page 215).
2. Slice the tomato with a serrated knife, arrange on plates, spread with pesto, top with the eggs, sprinkle with salt and pepper, and serve.

■ ■ ■ "MANNA FROM HEAVEN" BREAD WITH SMOKED SALMON PATÉ AND GREEN SALAD

The rich taste of this paté is quite lovely served on toast, and is well complemented with the tart and sweet salad. You can buy dulse flakes (a type of seaweed) at many health food stores.

SERVES 2

1 head Bibb lettuce, washed and dried

1 kiwi, sliced into half rounds

½ cup whole, raw pecans

2 tablespoons dulse (seaweed) flakes

CITRUS VINAIGRETTE (SEE RECIPE ON PAGE 232)

2 pieces "Manna from Heaven" bread, toasted

SMOKED SALMON PATÉ

4 ounces smoked salmon

2 tablespoons cream cheese

¼ cup fresh chopped basil

1 tablespoons fresh chopped dill

1 clove garlic

1 tablespoon chopped walnuts

1. Place the lettuce, kiwi, pecans, and dulse in a salad bowl.
2. Mix the citrus dressing.
3. Blend the salmon paté in a food processor.

4. Spread the salmon paté on Manna toast.
5. Toss the dressing with the salad and serve.

■ ■ ■ COUNTRY BUFFALO STEW

Here's a leaner version of a traditional favorite. Buffalo meat has a light, delicate flavor and is much lower in saturated fat than beef. Buffalo meat is sold at butchers, many supermarkets, and health food stores.

SERVES 2

1 pound buffalo stew meat

¼ cup flour

3 tablespoons extra virgin olive oil

2 medium onions, chopped

3 tablespoons chopped fresh rosemary

2 tablespoons chopped fresh thyme

1 quart beef stock

1 quart water

2 turnips, cut into chunks

5 celery stalks, chopped

5 carrots, cut into rounds

5 garlic cloves, chopped

½ head green cabbage, thinly sliced

1 teaspoon salt

¼ teaspoon black pepper

1 cup chopped fresh Italian parsley

1. Dredge the stew meat in flour, and discard the excess.
2. Heat the olive oil on medium heat in a large soup pot, add the buffalo meat and quickly brown.
3. Remove the pot from the heat, and place the meat in a separate bowl.
4. Add ¼ cup of the water to the pot, return to medium heat, add the onions, and cook until soft.

5. Add the herbs, the beef stock, the rest of the water, and the stew meat.
6. Bring to a boil and turn down to simmer, making sure that the meat is covered with liquid. Add a little water if necessary.
7. Simmer for 1½ hours, then add the vegetables, salt and black pepper, and simmer for another 20 to 30 minutes.
8. Serve garnished with parsley.

■ ■ ■ BLACK BEAN WRAP

With a spicy Mexican flair, this lunch will fill you up.

SERVES 2

BLACK BEAN SPREAD

    2 cups canned black soybeans, rinsed

    2 tablespoons tahini

    2 tablespoons extra virgin olive oil

    2 teaspoons ground cumin

    ¼ teaspoon ground coriander

    Pinch of cayenne

    Salt to taste

    2 low-carb La Tortilla Factory tortillas

    1 sliced avocado

    1 cup shredded lettuce

    1 carrot, grated

    ½ cup broccoli sprouts

1. Blend the ingredients for the black bean spread.
2. Spread the black bean spread on the tortillas ½ inch thick.
3. Lay the vegetables in a row on the tortillas, roll up, and serve.

■ ■ ■ MORE PIZZA

Try some different toppings on your pizza this time.

CRUST (SEE PIZZA WITH PESTO SAUCE, PAGE 263)
PESTO SAUCE

- 2 cups chopped fresh basil
- ½ cup olive oil
- ¼ cup walnuts
- 2 garlic cloves
- ⅓ cup grated Parmesan

- 1 boneless, skinless, chicken breast, sliced

TOPPING

- 2 tomatoes, thinly sliced
- 3 garlic cloves, chopped
- 1 tablespoon grated Parmesan
- ¼ cup chèvre

1. Preheat the grill.
2. Make the crust following the directions on page 263.
3. Blend the pesto.
4. Grill the chicken for 10 minutes on each side, and cut into thin slices.
5. Spread pesto on the baked crust, top with the tomatoes, garlic, Parmesan, chèvre, and chicken breasts.
6. Place back in the oven for 5 minutes.

▪ ▪ ▪ STUFFED PEPPERS

This dish is delicious and filling, but not heavy.

SERVES 2

2 large red bell peppers

1 medium onion, chopped

2 tablespoons olive oil

4 garlic cloves, minced

8 ounces ground turkey

6 ounces crushed tomatoes

1 tablespoon dried thyme

¼ cup chopped fresh basil

½ cup quinoa

Pinch of cayenne

Salt and pepper to taste

½ cup grated Parmesan

1. Preheat the oven to 350°F.
2. Fill a large saucepan three-quarters full with water and bring to a boil.
3. Cut the tops off each pepper and remove the seeds. When the water boils, drop each pepper in and cook for 5 minutes. Cool in cold water and put aside for later stuffing. Chop the red tops of the peppers.
4. Chop the onion and sauté in olive oil in a large, deep skillet. When translucent, add the peppers and sauté for 5 minutes.
5. Add the turkey and stir frequently until all the meat is brown, about 5 minutes.
6. Add the tomatoes and herbs, and cook for 10 to 15 minutes.
7. Cook the quinoa according to the directions on the box.
8. Add the cayenne, salt and pepper, grated Parmesan, and cooked quinoa to the stuffing mixture.
9. Stuff each pepper; top with more grated Parmesan. Bake at 350°F for 15 minutes.

■ ■ ■ FAUX MASHED POTATOES FROM TANGERINE

If you live anywhere near Los Angeles, check out Tangerine, a fabulous West Hollywood restaurant that offers some Rosedale Diet–approved dishes on their menu. This is one of my favorite recipes designed by Tangerine chef Bianca Simonian. It's great for people who crave mashed potatoes but don't want to fill up on starchy carbs.

SERVES 4

1 head cauliflower, leaves and stems removed, cut into quarters
2 tablespoons crème fraîche
½ stick, or 4 tablespoons, sweet butter
Salt and pepper to taste
½ cup almonds, finely ground in a blender
½ cup green onions, sliced thin

1. Preheat the oven to 400°F.
2. Boil water in a large sauce pan. Place the cauliflower in the boiling water and cook until soft.
3. Remove the cauliflower from the water, drain, and place in a bowl. Using a hand mixer, add crème fraîche, butter, salt, and pepper to the cauliflower. Whip until the cauliflower is smooth, or has the consistency of mashed potatoes.
4. Drain the cauliflower mixture in a finely meshed strainer to remove excess water. (If you don't have a strainer that is fine enough, strain the cauliflower through a coffee filter.)
5. By hand, mix in the nuts and green onions.
6. Grease a ring mold with butter. Add the cauliflower mixture.
7. Bake for 6 to 10 minutes, until the cauliflower is golden brown on top.

■ SNACKS

Grab a handful of these between meals.

Roasted Nuts

1. Make in batches to last for the week.
2. Preheat the oven to 400°F.
3. Mix the nuts and spices.
4. Roast on a baking sheet in the oven for 10 to 20 minutes.
5. Cool and store in the fridge, to avoid rancid oils.

TAMARI ALMONDS

2 cups almonds
1 tablespoon tamari
Pinch of cayenne

PUMPKIN PECANS

2 cups pecans
1 teaspoon melted ghee (clarified butter)
2 teaspoons pumpkin pie spice

SPICY CASHEWS

2 cups cashews
¼ teaspoon cayenne
½ teaspoon salt
¼ teaspoon cinnamon

Nutola

See recipe on page 218.

GINGER MACNUTS

2 cups macadamia nuts

¼ to ½ teaspoon powdered ginger

¼ teaspoon salt

CHAI NUTS

2 cups cashews

½ teaspoon cardamom

Pinch of cinnamon

Pinch of ginger

2 cups walnuts, dry-roasted in cast-iron pan

■ ■ ■ ALMONDS ALLA AUBERGINE

This recipe is from Spinelli's, a neighborhood grocer around the corner from my home. It is a great snack.

1 cup raw almonds

2 teaspoons olive oil

1½ teaspoon dried rosemary

1 teaspoon crushed chili pepper flakes

½ teaspoon semi-coarse sea salt

1. Preheat the oven to 200°F.
2. Spread the almonds onto a cookie sheet and roast for 45 minutes.
3. Remove the almonds from the oven and let them cool.
4. Place the almonds in a large bowl and add the olive oil, rosemary, pepper flakes, and salt. Mix well.
5. Store in an airtight container away from direct sunlight.

■ DIPS AND SPREADS

Make and keep in the fridge to snack on throughout the week.

■ ■ ■ STUFFED CELERY

3 celery stalks

STUFFING

¼ cup tahini

¼ cup almond butter

2 tablespoons flax oil

½ teaspoon cardamom

Pinch of cinnamon

Pinch of stevia powder

1 tablespoon chopped almonds

Chop the celery into thirds, fill with stuffing mixture, and sprinkle with almonds.

■ ■ ■ BASIL PESTO DIP

2 cups chopped fresh basil

½ cup extra virgin olive oil

¼ cup macadamia nuts

⅓ cup grated Parmesan

2 garlic cloves

Pinch of salt

Wasa crackers cut in thirds, sliced red bell peppers, carrot sticks, cucumber rounds, snap peas, broccoli florets, zucchini rounds

1. Mix the pesto in a food processor and place in a bowl.
2. Dip the cut vegetables, and munch.

■ ■ ■ CILANTRO PESTO DIP

2 cups chopped fresh cilantro
½ cup avocado oil
1 tablespoon lemon juice
¼ cup pine nuts
2 garlic cloves
Pinch of cayenne

1. Blend ingredients in a food processor and place in a bowl.
2. Serve with cut-up vegetables.

■ ■ ■ BLACK SOYBEAN DIP

2 cups black soybeans
2 tablespoons tahini (or feta)
2 tablespoons olive oil
2 teaspoons ground cumin
¼ teaspoon ground coriander
Salt to taste

1. Blend in a food processor.
2. Serve with crudités: peppers, carrots, cucumber, snap peas, broccoli, zucchini.

■ ■ ■ ROASTED RED BELL PEPPER DIP

1 red bell pepper
¼ cup pine nuts
1 garlic clove
2 tablespoons olive oil
1 teaspoon rosemary

1. Roast the pepper.
2. Blend all the ingredients in a food processor.

■ ■ ■ OLIVE TAPENADE

1 cup pitted Kalamata olives
2 tablespoons feta
2 tablespoons olive oil
½ cup fresh basil

1. Blend all the ingredients in a food processor.
2. Spread on "Manna from Heaven" bread; dip with cucumber rounds.

■ ■ ■ SALMON SPREAD

3 ounces smoked salmon
2 tablespoons low-fat cream cheese
¼ cup fresh basil
1 tablespoon fresh dill
1 garlic clove
1 tablespoon chopped walnuts

Blend all the ingredients in a food processor.

■ ■ ■ AVOCADO SPREAD

1 ripe avocado
1 garlic clove
1 teaspoon flax oil
1 tablespoon fresh lemon juice
¼ cup chopped fresh cilantro

Mix all the ingredients in a blender.

■ ■ ■ SUMMER HEALTH

Jena thanks Thea and Le Le for this recipe.
2 cups fresh parsley, stems and all
¼ cup olive oil
2 garlic cloves
⅛ cup grated Parmesan

Blend all the ingredients in a food processor.

■ ■ ■ HOMEMADE MAYONNAISE

SERVES 4

Put good fat back into your mayonnaise!
1 egg yolk
¼ cup avocado oil
1 tablespoon lemon juice
Pinch of cayenne

In a blender, mix the egg yolk and oil, then add the lemon juice and cayenne.

■ DESSERTS

■ ■ ■ RASPBERRY MOUSSE CAKE

Splenda is the only artificial sweetener that I allow on my diet, and only in very limited quantities. You can buy it at almost any supermarket.

SERVES 8

FILLING

- 2 small packages raspberries
- 1 package silken tofu
- 2 tablespoons fresh lemon juice
- 3 tablespoons Splenda

CRUST

- ½ cup cashews
- ½ cup almonds
- 4 tablespoons butter
- Pinch of nutmeg
- Pinch of cinnamon

1. Blend the filling in a food processor.
2. Blend the crust in the food processor, and press into a pie plate.
3. Pour the filling into the crust.
4. Chill for 3 hours. Serve.

■ ■ ■ BLUEBERRY CRUMBLE

This is a great dessert! You can use either Splenda, an artificial sweet-ener sold at supermarkets, or Stevia powder, a natural sweetener sold at health food stores.

SERVES 8

FILLING

    2 packages frozen blueberries
    1 tablespoon lemon juice
    1 teaspoon Stevia powder or Splenda
    1 teaspoon xanthan gum (found in health food stores)

TOPPING

    1 cup walnuts
    1 cup spelt flour
    ¼ teaspoon nutmeg
    Pinch of cinnamon
    4 tablespoons butter

1. Grease a glass pie plate with butter.
2. Mix the blueberry filling ingredients and place them in the bottom of the pie plate.
3. Blend the topping in a food processor.
4. Sprinkle the topping over the blueberry filling.
5. Bake for 40 minutes at 350°F.

■ ■ ■ TOFU CHOCOLATE MOUSSE

Tofu is a food of many disguises. It goes from "omeletes" to stir-fry with vegetables to chocolaty desserts without missing a beat.

SERVES 4–6

1 cake silken tofu

8 ounces Baker's chocolate, melted

2 teaspoons Stevia powder

1 tablespoon vanilla extract

Pinch of nutmeg

Pinch of cinnamon

1. Blend all the ingredients in a food processor.
2. Spoon into wineglasses.
3. Chill for 2 hours.
4. Serve topped with raspberries.

■ ■ ■ BERRIES AND CREAM

Good enough for an elegant dinner party

SERVES 2

⅓ cup strawberries

⅓ cup blueberries

⅓ cup blackberries

½ cup cream

Mix the berries in a bowl, top with cream, and serve.

■ ■ ■ RICOTTA CHEESECAKE

This recipe and the one that follows (French Silk Pie) are two very popular desserts served at Tangerine, a fabulous West Hollywood restaurant where some Rosedale Diet–approved menu items are available to the customers.

NUT CRUST

　　2 cups nuts (of your choice)

　　3 tablespoons butter, softened

1. Place the nuts in a food processor and blend them until they are powder-like.
2. Add the butter.
3. By hand, form a ¼"-thick nut crust inside a pan.

CAKE

　　1 container (15 ounces) ricotta cheese

　　⅓ cup Splenda

　　¼ cup half-and-half

　　2 tablespoons flour (you can use the nut powder)

　　½ tablespoon vanilla

　　2 eggs

1. Preheat the oven to 350°F.
2. Blend together the ricotta, Splenda, half-and-half, flour/nut powder, and vanilla.
3. Add the eggs and mix everything until blended.
4. Pour the mixture into the nut crust.
5. Bake at 350°F for 45–50 minutes.
6. Refrigerate for 3 hours or overnight.

TIP: You can top the cake with fresh fruits and berries.

■ ■ ■ FRENCH SILK PIE

NUT CRUST

　　See Ricotta Cheesecake, above.

PIE

4 cups (1 pound) butter, softened

1⅓ cups Splenda

8 ounces dark (unsweetened) chocolate, melted, then cooled to room temperature

4 teaspoons vanilla

2 cups egg product (e.g., Egg Beaters, egg whites)

1 cup whipping cream, whipped

1. Cream together butter and Splenda.
2. Mix the chocolate with vanilla.
3. Add the egg product and mix everything with a hand mixer until it is smooth and thick like a mousse.
4. Pour the mixture into the nut crust and refrigerate for 1–2 hours.
5. Top the pie with whipped cream.

··· Product Information

To order "Manna from Heaven" bread, call the Julian Bakery, La Jolla, CA, at 800-98BREAD.

La Tortilla Factory low-carb tortillas are available at many health food stores and can be ordered from their Web site at www.LaTortilla Factory.com.

For more information on Dr. Rosedale's supplement line, contact:
Rosedale Metabolics
P.O. Box 370508
Denver, CO 80237-0508
303-790-8766
Or visit his Web site at www.rosedalemetabolics.com.

To contact Jena Latham of Fresh Cuisine, call 808-281-6551.

The following laboratories can test leptin level and perform the medical tests mentioned in this book:

Esoterix Laboratory Services
800-444-9111
Or visit their Web site at www.esoterix.com

Quest Diagnostics
800-777-8448
Or visit their Web site at www.questdiagnostics.com

Labcorp
800-331-1843
Or visit their Web site at www.labcorp.com

··· References

▪ LEPTIN; GENERAL

Ahima R. S. Role of leptin in the neuroendocrine response to fasting. Nature 1996, Vol. 382, 250–52.

Ainsworth, Claire. Love That Fat, *New Scientist* magazine, Vol. 167, Iss. 2256, p. 36.

Baile, Clifton A., Regulation of metabolism and body fat mass by leptin. *Annual Review of Nutrition,* 2000, Vol. 20, 105–27.

Campfield, L. Arthur. Central mechanisms responsible for the actions of OB protein (leptin) on food intake, metabolism and body energy storage. *Neuroendocrinology of Leptin,* Ur, E. (ed). Karger, 2000, Vol 26, pp. 12–20.

Gura, Trisha. Is leptin a "thrifty" hormone in muscle and fat? *Science,* Vol. 287, p. 1739.

Harris, Ruth B. S. Leptin—much more than a satiety signal. *Annual Review of Nutrition,* 2000, Vol. 20, 45–75.

Havel, P. J. Control of energy homeostasis and insulin action by adipocyte hormones: leptin, acylation stimulating protein, and adiponectin. *Current Opinion in Lipidology,* 2002, Vol. 13, Iss.1, 51–59.

Kawai, Kirio. Leptin as a modulator of sweet taste sensitivities in mice. *Proceedings of the National Academy of Science,* 2000, Vol. 97, Iss. 20, 11044–49.

Pinto, S. Rapid rewiring of arcuate nucleus feeding circuits by leptin. *Science*, Vol. 304, 2004, 110–15.

Rosenbaum, M. and Rudolph L. Leibel. Leptin: A molecule integrating somatic energy stores, energy expenditure and fertility. *Trends in Endocrinology and Metabolism*, Vol. 9, Iss. 3, 1998.

Travis, J. Hormone signals the death of fat cells. *Science News,* Vol. 153, Iss. 5, 70.

Unger H. Regulation of fatty acid homeostasis in cells: Novel role of leptin. *Proceedings of the National Academy of Science USA*, 1999, Vol. 96, 2327–32.

▪ DIET AND LEPTIN CONCENTRATION

Agus, M. S. Dietary composition and physiologic adaptations to energy restriction. *American Journal of Clinical Nutrition,* 2000, Vol. 71, Iss. 4, 901–07.

Ainslie, D. A. Short-term, high-fat diets lower circulating leptin concentrations in rats. *American Journal of Clinical Nutrition,* 2000, Vol. 71, 438–42.

Boado, R. J. Up-regulation of blood-brain barrier short-form leptin receptor gene products in rats fed a high fat diet. *Journal of Neurochemistry,* 1998, Vol. 71, Iss.4, 1761–64.

Mueller, W. M. Evidence that glucose metabolism regulates leptin secretion from cultured rat adipocytes. *Endocrinology,* 1998, Vol. 139, Iss. 2, 551–58.

Torgerson, J. A low serum leptin level at baseline and a large early decline in leptin predict a large 1-year weight reduction in energy-restricted obese humans. *Journal of Clinical Endocrinology and Metabolism,* 1999, Vol. 84, 4197–4203.

Wadden, T. A. Short and long-term changes in serum leptin in dieting obese women: effects of caloric restriction and weight loss. *Journal of Clinical Endocrinology and Metabolism,* 1998, Vol. 83 Iss. 1, 214–18.

▪ LEPTIN: INSULIN SENSITIVITY, GLUCOSE AND DIABETES

Barzilai, N. Interaction between aging and syndrome X: new insights on the pathophysiology of fat distribution. *Annals of the New York Academy of Science,* 1999, Vol. 892, 58–72.

Cases, J. A. The regulation of body fat distribution and the modulation of insulin action. *International Journal of Obesity and Related Metabolic Disorders,* 2000, Suppl. 4, S63–66.

Kieffer, T. J. The adipoinsular axis: effects of leptin on pancreatic b-cells. *American Journal of Physiology, Endocrinology and Metabolism*, 2000, Vol. 278: E1–E14.

Sweeney, G. High leptin levels acutely inhibit insulin-stimulated glucose uptake without affecting glucose transporter 4 translocation in 16 rat skeletal muscle cells. *Endocrinology*, 2001, Vol. 142, Iss. 11, 4806–12.

■ LEPTIN AND THE SYMPATHETIC NERVOUS SYSTEM

Figlewicz, D. P. Adiposity signals and food reward: expanding the CNS roles of insulin and leptin. *American Journal of Physiology—Regulatory, Integrative and Comparative Physiology*, 2003, Vol. 284, R882–R892.

■ LEPTIN AND THYROID

Flier, J. S. Leptin, nutrition, and the thyroid: the why, the wherefore, and the wiring. *The Journal of Clinical Investigation*, 2000, Vol. 105, Iss. 7, 859.

Harris M. Transcriptional regulation of the thyrotropin-releasing hormone gene by leptin and melanocortin signaling. *The Journal of Clinical Investigation*, 2001, Vol. 107, 111–120.

■ LEPTIN AND OSTEOPOROSIS

Ducy P. The osteoblast: A sophisticated fibroblast under central surveillance. *Science,* 2000, Vol. 289, 1502–04.

Karsenty, G. The Central Regulation of Bone Remodeling. *Trends in Endocrinology and Metabolism*, 2000, Vol. 11, Iss. 10, 437–439.

■ CALCIUM AND BONE

Beckman, M. Dense matter. *Science of Aging. Knowledge Environment,* 2003, Vol. 48, pp. nw164.

Michaelsson, K. Dietary calcium and vitamin D intake in relation to osteoporotic fracture risk. *Bone*, 2002, Vol. 32, 694–703.

■ LEPTIN AND ABDOMINAL FAT

Barzilai, N. Interaction between aging and syndrome X: new insights on the pathophysiology of fat distribution. *Annals of the New York Academy of Science,* 1999, Vol. 892, 58–72.

Cnop, M. The concurrent accumulation of intra-abdominal and subcutaneous fat explains the association between insulin resistance and plasma leptin concentrations. *Diabetes,* 2002, Vol. 51, Iss. 4, 1005–15.

Friedman, J. Fat in all the wrong places. Nature, 2002, Vol. 415, Iss. 17, 268–269.

■ AGING: LEPTIN AND INSULIN CONNECTION

Bartke, A. Mutations prolong life in flies; implications for aging in mammals. *Trends in Endocrinology and Metabolism,* 2001, Vol. 12, Iss. 6, 233.

Chiba, T. Anti-aging effects of caloric restriction: Involvement of neuroendocrine adaptation by peripheral signaling. *Microscopy Research and Technique,* 2002, Vol. 59, Iss. 4, 317–24.

Heininger, K. Aging is a deprivation syndrome driven by a germ-soma conflict. *Ageing Research Reviews,* 2002, Vol. 1, 481–536.

Nelson, D. W. Insulin worms its way into the spotlight. *Genes and Development,* 2003, Vol. 17, 813–18.

Overton, J. M. Central leptin infusion attenuates the cardiovascular and metabolic effects of fasting in rats. *Hypertension,* 2001, Vol. 37, Iss. 2, 663–69.

Partridge, L. Mechanisms of aging: public or private? *Nature Reviews, Genetics,* Vol. 3, Iss. 3, 173.

Shimokawa, I. Leptin and anti-aging action of caloric restriction. *The Journal of Nutrition, Health and Aging,* 2001, Vol. 5, 43–48.

———. Leptin signaling and aging: insight from caloric restriction. *Mechanisms of Ageing and Development,* 2001, Vol. 122, Iss. 14, 1511–19.

■ LEPTIN AND REPRODUCTION

Caprio, M. Leptin in reproduction. *Trends in Endocrinology and Metabolism,* 2001, Vol. 12, Iss. 2, 65–72.

Holness, M. J. At the cutting edge; current concepts concerning the role of leptin in reproductive function. *Molecular and Cellular Endocrinology,* 1999, Vol. 157, 11–20.

Kiess, W. A role for leptin in sexual maturation and puberty? *Hormone Research,* 1999, Vol. 51, supp. 3, 55–63.

Matkovic, V. Leptin is inversely related to age at menarche in human females. *Journal of Clinical Endocrinology and Metabolism,* 1997, Vol. 82, 3239–45.

▪ LEPTIN; HEART AND VASCULAR DISEASE

Aizawa-Abe, M. Pathophysiological role of leptin in obesity-related hypertension. *Journal of Clinical Investigation,* 2000, Vol. 105, Iss. 9, 1243–52.

Barouch, L. A. Disruption of leptin signaling contributes to cardiac hypertrophy independently of body weight in mice. *Circulation,* 2003, Vol. 108, Iss. 6, 754–59.

Parhami, F. Leptin enhances the calcification of vascular cells: artery wall as a target of leptin. *Circulation Research,* 2001, Vol. 88, Iss. 9, 954–60.

Wallace, A. M. Plasma leptin and the risk of cardiovascular disease in the west of Scotland coronary prevention study (WOSCOPS). *Circulation,* 2001, Vol. 104, 3052–56.

▪ LEPTIN AND AUTOIMMUNITY

Kuchroo, V. K. Immunology: Fast and feel good? *Nature,* 2003, Vol. 422, 27–28.

Matarese, G. Leptin accelerates autoimmune diabetes in female NOD mice. *Diabetes,* 2002, Vol. 51, Iss. 5, 1356–61.

Sanna, V. Leptin surge precedes onset of autoimmune encephalomyelitis and correlates with development of pathogenic T cell responses. *Journal of Clinical Investigation,* 2003, Vol. 111, 241–50.

▪ W-3 FATTY ACIDS AND LEPTIN

Reseland, J. E. Reduction of leptin gene expression by dietary polyunsaturated fatty acids. *Journal of Lipid Research,* 2001, Vol. 42, Iss. 5, 743–50.

■ CANCER: DIET, LEPTIN, INSULIN, AND GLUCOSE

Anisimov, V. N. Insulin/IGF-1 signaling pathway driving aging and cancer as a target for pharmacological intervention. *Experimental Gerontology,* 2003, Vol. 38, Iss. 10, 1041–49.

Okumura, M. Leptin and high glucose stimulate cell proliferation in MCF-7 human breast cancer cells: reciprocal involvement of PKC-alpha and PPAR expression. *Biochimica et Biophysical Acta,* 2002, Vol. 1592, Iss. 2, 107–16.

Seyfried, T. N. Role of glucose and ketone bodies in the metabolic control of experimental brain cancer. *British Journal of Cancer,* 2003, Vol. 89, Iss. 7, 1375–82.

■ CALORIC RESTRICTION AND INCREASED LONGEVITY

Blüher, M. Extended longevity in mice lacking the insulin receptor in adipose tissue. *Science,* 2003, Vol. 299, Iss. 24, 572–74.

Duffy, P. H. Effect of chronic caloric restriction on physiological variables related to energy metabolism in the male Fischer 344 rat. *Mechanisms of Aging and Development,* 1989, Vol. 48, Iss. 2, 117–33.

Fernandez-Galaz, C. Long-term food restriction prevents aging-associated central leptin resistance in wistar rats. *Diabetologia,* 2002, Vol. 45, Iss. 7, 997–1003.

Hansen, B. C. Symposium: Calorie restriction: Effects on body composition, insulin signaling and aging. *Journal of Nutrition,* 2001, Vol. 131, 900S– 902S.

Hursting, S. D. Calorie restriction, aging, and cancer prevention: Mechanisms of action and applicability to humans. *Annual Review of Medicine,* 2003, Vol. 54, 131–52.

Mattison, J. A. Endocrine effects of dietary restriction and aging: The National Institute of Aging Study. *Journal of Anti-Aging Medicine,* 2001, Vol. 4, Iss. 3, 215–24.

Roth, G. S. Biomarkers of caloric restriction may predict longevity in humans. *Science,* 2002, Vol. 297, Iss. 2, 811.

Roth, G. S. Effects of reduced energy intake on the biology of aging: the primate model. *European Journal of Clinical Nutrition,* 2000, Vol. 54, Iss. S3, S15–S20.

■ BENEFITS OF EATING GOOD FATS

Greene, A. E., Perspectives on the metabolic management of epilepsy through dietary reduction of glucose and elevation of ketone bodies. *Journal of Neurochemistry,* 2003, Vol. 86, 529–37.

Iossa, S. Skeletal muscle oxidative capacity in rats fed high-fat diet. *International Journal of Obesity and Related Metabolic Disorders,* 2002, Vol. 26, Iss. 1, 65–72.

Louheranta, A. M. Association of the fatty acid profile of serum lipids with glucose and insulin metabolism during 2 fat-modified diets in subjects with impaired glucose tolerance. *American Journal of Clinical Nutrition,* 2002, Vol. 76, 331–37.

Magnan C. Lipid infusion lowers sympathetic nervous activity and leads to increased beta-cell responsiveness to glucose. *Journal of Clinical Investigation,* 1999, Vol. 103, Iss. 3, 413–19.

Marckmann, P. Fishing for heart protection. *American Journal of Clinical Nutrition,* 2003, Vol. 78, 1–2.

McCargar L. J. Influence of dietary carbohydrate-to-fat ratio on whole body nitrogen retention and body composition in adult rats. *Journal of Nutrition,* 1989, Vol. 119, Iss. 9, 1240–45.

Mlekusch, W. The life-shortening effect of reduced physical activity is abolished by a fat rich diet. *Mechanisms of Aging and Development,* 1998, Vol. 105, 61–73.

Reed, D. R. Enhanced acceptance and metabolism of fats by rats fed a high-fat diet. *American Journal of Physiology,* 1991, Vol. 261, Iss. 5, Pt. 2, R1084–88.

Seyfried, T. N. Role of glucose and ketone bodies in the metabolic control of experimental brain cancer. *Br J Cancer,* 2003, Vol. 89, Iss. 7, 1375–82.

Smith, S. R. Fat and carbohydrate balances during adaptation to a high-fat diet. *American Journal of Clinical Nutrition,* 2000, Vol. 71, 450–57.

■ SATURATED FAT: DANGERS OF EXCESS

Montell, E. L. DAG accumulation from saturated fatty acids desensitizes insulin stimulation of glucose uptake in muscle cells. *American Journal of Physiology—Endocrinology and Metabolism,* 2001, Vol. 280, 229–37.

Wang, L. Plasma fatty acid composition and incidence of diabetes in middle-aged adults: the Atherosclerosis Risk in Communities (ARIC) Study. *American Journal of Clinical Nutrition*, 2003, Vol. 78, 91–98.

■ BENEFITS OF LIMITED PROTEIN

Bandyopadhyay, B. C. Hypothalamic GABA-ergic activity and T cell proliferation in aged mammal: effect of dietary protein. *Neurochem International*, 1998, Vol. 32, Iss. 2, 191–96.

De, A. K. Some biochemical parameters of aging in relation to dietary protein. *Mechanisms of Aging and Development*, Vol. 21, 1983, 37–48.

Fleming, R. M. The effect of high-protein diets on coronary blood flow. *Angiology*, 2000, Vol. 51, Iss. 10, 817–26.

Gannon, M. C. Effect of protein ingestion on the glucose appearance rate in people with type 2 diabetes. *The Journal of Clinical Endocrinology and Metabolism*, Vol. 86, Iss. 3, 1040–47.

Lariviere, F. Effects of dietary protein restriction on glucose and insulin metabolism in normal and diabetic humans. *Metabolism*, 1994, Vol. 43, Iss. 4, 462–67.

Linn, T. Effect of dietary protein intake on insulin secretion and glucose metabolism in insulin-dependent diabetes mellitus. *Clinical Endocrinology and Metabolism*, 1996, Vol. 81, Iss. 11, 3938–43.

Westerterp, K. R. Diet induced thermogenesis measured over 24 hours in a respiration chamber: effect of diet composition. *International Journal of Obesity and Related Metabolic Disorder*, 1999, Vol. 23, Iss. 3, 287–92.

■ SUPPLEMENTS

Anderson, R. A. Elevated intakes of supplemental chromium improve glucose and insulin variables in individuals with type 2 diabetes. *Diabetes*, 1997, Vol. 146, 1786–91.

Binkley, N. C. A high phylloquinone intake is required to achieve maximal osteocalcin—carboxylation. *American Journal of Clinical Nutrition*, 2002, Vol. 76, 1055–60.

Engelen, W. Effects of long-term supplementation with moderate pharmacologic doses of vitamin E are saturable and reversible in patients with type 1 diabetes. *American Journal of Clinical Nutrition*, 2000, Vol. 72, 1142–44.

Killilea, L. J. Delaying the mitochondrial decay of aging. *Proceedings of the National Academy of Science USA,* 2002, Vol. 99, 1876–81.

Wang, S. Effects of chromium and fish oil on insulin resistance and leptin resistance in obese developing rats. *Wei Sheng Yan Jiu,* 2001, Iss. 5, 284–86.

···General Index

···Recipe Index

A

almonds:
  alla aubergine, 280
  in arugula salad, 240–41
  in broccoli soup, 261
  in faux mashed potatoes from
    Tangerine, 278
  in mung dal soup and mesclun salad,
    229–30
  in nutola, 218
  in raspberry mousse cake, 285
  sauce, lemony, tofu and broccoli in,
    247–48
  smoothie with, 223
  in spicy chicken salad, 234
  tamari, 279
apple:
  in mung dal soup and mesclun salad,
    229–30
  in spicy chicken salad, 234

artichoke hearts, in pizza with pesto
    sauce, 263–64
arugula:
  in Maui salad, 226
  salad, 240–41
asparagus:
  fresh, dilled salmon and, 217
  salmon cakes with, 234–35
  in salmon salad, 218–19
  soup and deviled eggs, 236–37
avocado:
  in berry good salad, 256
  in black bean wrap, 275
  in eggs "benefit," 215
  in lobster tails and seaweed salad,
    222–23
  in mung dal soup and mesclun salad,
    229–30
  in romaine salad à la Ron, 241–42
  and smoked salmon toasts,
    225–26
  spread, 284

Z